Al Pruitt 08'

David J. Goldberg (Ed.)

Laser Dermatology

David J. Goldberg (Ed.)

Laser Dermatology

With 108 Figures and 15 Tables

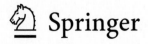 Springer

Dr. David J. Goldberg
Skin Laser & Surgery Specialists
of New York and New Jersey
20 Prospect Avenue
Suite 702
Hackensack, NJ 07601
USA

ISBN 3-540-21277-9 Springer Berlin Heidelberg New York

Library of Congress Control Number: 2004110370

Springer is a part of Springer Science+Business Media

springeronline.com

© Springer-Verlag Berlin Heidelberg 2005
Printed in The Netherlands

Editor: Marion Philipp
Desk Editor: Irmela Bohn
Production: ProEdit GmbH, 69126 Heidelberg, Germany
Cover: Frido Steinen-Broo, EStudio Calamar, Spain
Typesetting: Satz-Druck-Service, 69181 Leimen, Germany

Printed on acid-free paper   24/3180 Re   5 4 3 2 1   SPIN 12175840

Preface

The continual array of laser technology throughout the world has been nothing short of miraculous. Over the last fifteen years, this field has continued to grow and expand with the appearance of new technology. This book represents the most up-to-date description of the latest in laser and light-source technology. All the chapters are written by leading experts from both North America and Europe. After a chapter describing our latest understanding of laser physics, which also covers safety aspects, chapters are dedicated to laser treatment of vascular lesions, pigmented lesions and tattoos, unwanted hair, and ablative and non-ablative resurfacing and treatment for medical purposes. Each chapter begins with the core concepts. These basic points are followed by a history of the use of lasers for the cutaneous problem under discussion, currently available technology, and indications and contraindications. Each author then provides an example of his/her consent form and approaches to personal treatment.

What has become clear is that a significant understanding of lasers and light sources is required for optimum use of this technology. A basic understanding of laser physics is also fundamental to good laser treatment. Laser safety and minimizing risk to patients is at least as important as an understanding of laser physics. When these concepts, so clearly described in Chap. 1, are understood cutaneous laser technology can be safely and successfully used for a variety of purposes.

A wide variety of cutaneous vascular disorders can be successfully treated with modern lasers. The pulsed dye laser has enabled treatment of cutaneous vessels by following the principle of selective photothermolysis, a simple physics concept seen throughout laser dermatology. The pulsed dye laser is the most effective laser for treatment of port wine stains but purpura limits its acceptability by patients for more cosmetic indications. Both facial and leg vein telangiectasia can also be treated with lasers. Other cutaneous disorders such as psoriasis, warts and scars can be improved by targeting the lesion's cutaneous vessels with appropriate lasers. Chapter 2 describes our latest understanding of the laser treatment of vascular lesions.

When considering treatment of pigmented lesions, accurate diagnosis of the pigmented lesion is mandatory before laser treatment. For some pigmented lesions, laser treatment may even be the only treatment option. Tattoos respond well to Q-switched lasers. Amateur and traumatic tattoos respond more readily to treatment than do professional tattoos. Cosmetic tattoos should be approached with caution. Treatment of melanocytic nevi remains controversial, but worth pursuing. Chapter 3 describes our latest understanding of the laser treatment of pigmented lesions and tattoos.

A wide variety of lasers can now induce permanent changes in unwanted hair. Hair-removal lasers are distinguished not only by their emitted wavelengths, but also by their delivered pulse duration, peak fluence, spot size delivery system and associated cooling. Nd:YAG lasers, with effective cooling, are the safest approach for treatment of darker skin. Despite this, complications arising from laser hair removal are more common in darker skin types. Laser treatment of non-pigmented hair remains a challenge. Chapter 4 describes our latest understanding of the laser treatment of unwanted hair

Ablative and non-ablative laser resurfacing lead to improvement of photodamaged skin.

Ablative laser resurfacing produces a significant wound, but long lasting clinical results.

Non-ablative resurfacing is cosmetically elegant, but generally leads to subtle improvement only. Visible light non-ablative devices lead to a lessening of erythema and superficial pigmentary skin changes. Mid-infrared laser devices promote better skin quality and skin toning. Chapter 5 describes our latest understanding of ablative and non-ablative laser resurfacing.

Lasers and light sources have become more commonplace in the treatment of dermatological medical diseases. Topical ALA and adjunct light-source therapy (ALA-PDT) is a proven photodynamic therapy for actinic keratoses and superficial non-melanoma skin cancers. ALA-PDT, using a variety of vascular lasers, blue-light sources, and intense pulsed light sources, is also now being used to treat the signs of photoaging. PDT can also be useful therapy for acne vulgaris. Newer lasers and light sources are also now being used to treat psoriasis vulgaris, vitiligo, other disorders of pigmentation, and hypopigmented stretch marks. Chapter 6 describes our latest understanding of photodynamic therapy and the treatment of medical dermatological conditions.

January 2005
David J. Goldberg

Contents

List of Contributors

Christine C. Dierickx, MD
Director Skin and Laser Surgery Center
Beukenlaan 52
2850 Boom
Belgium
e-mail: mail@cDierickx.be

Michael H. Gold, MD
Gold Skin Care Center
2000 Richard Jones Road
Suite 220
Nashville
TN 37215
USA
e-mail: drgold@goldskincare.com

David J. Goldberg, MD
Clinical Professor
Director of Laser Research
Department of Dermatology
Mount Sinai School of Medicine
Director of Dermatologic Surgery
UMDNJ-New Jersey Medical School
Director. Skin Laser & Surgery Specialists
of NY/NJ
e-mail: drdavidgoldberg@skinandlasers.com

Mussarrat Hussain, MD
Research Assistant
Skin Laser & Surgery Specialists of NY/NJ

Suzanne L. Kilmer, MD
3835 J Street
Sacramento
CA 95816
USA
e-mail: skilmer@skinlasers.com

Sean W. Lanigan, MD, FRCP, DCH
Consultant Dermatologist
Lasercare Clinics
City Hospital
Dudley Road
Birmingham
B18 7QH
UK
e-mail: Sean.lanigan@swbh.nhs.uk

Natalie Semchyshyn, MD
3835 J Street
Sacramento
CA 95816
USA
e-mail: nsemchyshyn@skinlasers.com

Ronald G. Wheeland, MD, FACP
Professor and Chief
Section of Dermatology
University of Arizona
e-mail: wheeland@email. arizona.edu

Basic Laser Physics and Safety

Ronald G. Wheeland

Core Messages

- A significant understanding of lasers and light sources is required for optimal use of these technologies
- A basic understanding of laser physics is at the core of good laser treatments
- Laser safety and minimizing patient risk is at least as important as an understanding of laser physics.

History

What Is Light?

Light is a very complex system of radiant energy that is composed of waves and energy packets known as photons. It is arranged into the electromagnetic spectrum (EMS) according to the length of those waves. The distance between two successive troughs or crests of these waves, measured in meters, determines the *wavelength*. For the visible portion of the EMS, the wavelength determines the color of the laser light. The number of wave crests (or troughs) that pass a given point in a second determines the *frequency* for each source of EMS energy. The wavelength and frequency of light are inversely related to one another. Thus, shorter wavelengths of light have higher frequencies and more energetic photons than longer wavelengths of light which have lower frequencies and less energetic photons.

■ When Was Light First Used for Medical Purposes?

One must go back to about 4000 B.C. in ancient Egypt to find the earliest recorded use of light. It was at that time that sunlight coupled with a topical photosensitizer, like parsley or other herbs containing psoralen, to help repigment individuals suffering from vitiligo, where the skin becomes depigmented through a presumed autoimmune reaction. In Europe in the 19th century, sunlight was used as a treatment for cutaneous tuberculosis. However, it wasn't until 1961 that Dr. Leon Goldman, a dermatologist at the University of Cincinnati, first employed a ruby laser for the removal of tattoos and other pigmented cutaneous lesions. For his continuous efforts in promoting the use of lasers for medical purposes and for co-founding the American Society for Laser Medicine and Surgery, Dr. Goldman (Goldman et al. 1963) has been called the "Father of Lasers in Medicine and Surgery." Since those earliest days, many physicians in different specialties have played key roles in the advancement of the use of lasers in medicine such that today most specialties use lasers in either diagnosing or treating a number of different disorders and diseases (Wheeland 1995).

■ Who Invented the Laser?

Professor Albert Einstein (Einstein 1917) published all of the necessary formulas and theoretical concepts to build a laser in his 1917 treatise called The Quantum Theory of Radiation. In this treatise, he described the interaction of atoms and molecules with electromagnetic energy in terms of the spontaneous absorption and emission of energy. By applying principles of thermodynamics he concluded that stimulated emission of energy was also possible. However, it wasn't until 1959 that Drs. Charles H. Townes and Arthur L. Schalow (Schalow and Townes 1958) developed the first instrument based on those concepts, known as the *MASER* (*M*icrowave *A*mplification through the *S*timulated *E*mission of *R*adiation). Then, in 1960, the first true laser, a ruby laser, was operated by Dr. Theodore H. Maiman (Maiman 1960). The development of additional lasers occurred rapidly, with the helium-neon laser appearing in 1961, the argon laser in 1962, the carbon dioxide and Nd:YAG laser in 1964, the dye laser in 1966, the excimer laser in 1975, the copper vapor laser in 1981, and the gold vapor laser in 1982.

What Is a Laser?

The word "LASER" is an acronym that stands for *L*ight *A*mplification by the *S*timulated *E*mission of *R*adiation. For this reason, a laser is not just an instrument but also a physical process of amplification (Table 1.1). The last word in the acronym, "radiation," is a common source of patient anxiety since it is associated with the high energy ionizing radiation often associated with cancer radiotherapy. However, in the case of lasers, the word is employed to describe how the laser light is propagated through space as "radiant" waves. Patients should be assured that all currently approved medical lasers are incapable of ionizing tissue and have none of the risks associated with the radiation used in cancer therapy.

All lasers are composed of the same four primary components. These include the *laser medium* (usually a solid, liquid, or gas), the *optical cavity* or resonator which surrounds the laser medium and contains the amplification process, the *power supply* or "pump" that excites the atoms and creates population inversion, and a *delivery system* (usually a fiber optic or articulating arm with mirrored joints) to precisely deliver the light to the target.

Lasers are usually named for the *medium* contained within their optical cavity (Table 1.2). The gas lasers consist of the argon, excimers, copper vapor, helium-neon, krypton, and carbon dioxide devices. One of the most common liquid lasers contains a fluid with rhodamine dye and is used in the pulsed dye laser. The solid lasers are represented by the ruby, neodymium:yttrium-aluminum-garnet (Nd:YAG), alexandrite, erbium, and diode lasers. All of these devices are used to clinically treat a wide variety of conditions and disorders based on their wavelength, nature of their pulse, and energy.

The excitation mechanism, i. e., power supply or "pump," is a necessary component of every laser in order to generate excited electrons and create population inversion (Arndt and Noe 1982). This can be accomplished by direct electrical current, optical stimulation by another laser (argon), radiofrequency excitation, white light from a flashlamp, or even (rarely) chemical reactions that either make or break chemical bonds to release energy, as in the hydrogen-fluoride laser.

To understand stand how laser light is created it is important to recall the structure of an atom. All atoms are composed of a central nucleus surrounded by electrons that occupy discrete energy levels or orbits around the nucleus and give the atom a stable configuration (Fig. 1.1). When an atom spontaneously absorbs a photon of light, the outer orbital electrons briefly move to a higher energy orbit, which is an unstable configuration (Fig. 1.2). This configuration is very evanescent and the atom quickly releases a photon of light spontaneously so the electrons can return to their normal, lower energy, but stable inner orbital configuration (Fig. 1.3). Under normal circumstances, this spontaneous absorption and release of light occurs in a disorganized and random fashion and results in the production of *incoherent* light.

When an external source of energy is supplied to a laser cavity containing the laser medium, usually in the form of electricity, light, microwaves, or even a chemical reaction, the resting atoms are stimulated to drive their electrons to unstable, higher energy, outer orbits. When more atoms exist in this unstable high energy configuration than in their usual resting configuration, a condition known as *population inversion* is created, which is necessary for the subsequent step in light amplification (Fig. 1.4).

Table 1.1. Laser terminology

Absorption	The transformation of radiant energy to another form of energy (usually heat) by interacting with matter
Coherence	All waves are in phase with one another in both time and space
Collimation	All waves are parallel to one another with little divergence or convergence
Electromagnetic radiation	A complex system of radiant energy composed of waves and energy bundles that is organized according to the length of the propagating wave
Energy	The product of power (watts) and pulse duration (seconds) which is expressed in joules
Extinction length	The thickness of a material necessary to absorb 98% of the incident energy
Focus	The exact point at which the laser energy is at peak power
Irradiance (power density)	The quotient of incident laser power on a unit surface area, expressed as watts/cm²
Joule	A unit of energy which equals one watt-second
Laser	An instrument that generates a beam of light of a single wavelength or color that is both highly collimated and coherent; an acronym that stands for light amplification by the stimulated emission of radiation
Laser medium	A material or substance of solid, liquid, or gaseous nature that is capable of producing laser light due to stimulated electron transition from an unstable high energy orbit to a lower one with release of collimated, coherent, monochromatic light
Meter	A unit length based on the spectrum of krypton-86; frequently subdivided into millimeters (10^{-3} m), micrometers (10^{-6} m), and nanometers (10^{-9} m)
Monochromatic	Light energy emitted from a laser optical cavity of only a single wavelength
Optically pumped laser	A laser where electrons are excited by the absorption of light energy from an external source
Photoacoustic effect	The ability of Q-switched laser light to generate a rapidly moving wave within living tissue that destroys melanin pigment and tattoo ink particles
Population inversion	The state present within the laser optical cavity (resonator) where more atoms exist in unstable high energy levels than their normal resting energy levels
Power	The rate at which energy is emitted from a laser
Power density (irradiance)	The quotient of incident laser power on a unit surface area, expressed as watts/cm²
Pump	The electrical, optical, radiofrequency or chemical excitation that provides energy to the laser medium
Q-switch	An optical device (Pockels cell) that controls the storage or release of laser energy from a laser optical cavity
Reflectance	The ratio of incident power to absorbed power by a given medium
Scattering	Imprecise absorption of laser energy by a biologic system resulting in a diffuse effect on tissue
Selective photothermolysis	A concept used to localize thermal injury to a specific target based on its absorption characteristics, the wavelength of light used, the duration of the pulse, and the amount of energy delivered
Thermomodulation	The ability of low energy light to upregulate certain cellular biologic activities without producing an injury
Transmission	The passage of laser energy through a biologic tissue without producing any effect

Amplification of light occurs in the optical cavity or resonator of the laser. The resonator typically consists of an enclosed cavity that allows the emitted photons of light to reflect back and forth from one mirrored end of the chamber to the other many times until a sufficient intensity has been developed for complete amplification to occur. Through a complex process of absorption and emission of photons of energy, the prerequisite for the development of a laser beam of light has been met and amplification occurs. The photons are then allowed to escape through a small perforation in the partially reflective mirror. The emerging beam of light has three unique characteristics that allow it to be delivered to the appropriate target by fiber optics or an articulated arm.

■ What Are the Unique Characteristics of Laser Light?

By stimulating the emission of light from a laser, laser light has three unique characteristics that differentiate it from nonlaser light. The first of these characteristics is that laser light is

Table 1.2. Types of lasers

Name	Type	Wavelength
ArFl	Excimer	193 nm
KrCl	Excimer	222 nm
KrFl	Excimer	248 nm
XeCl	Excimer	308 nm
XeFl	Excimer	351 nm
Argon	Gas	488 and 514 nm
Copper vapor	Gas	511 and 578 nm
Krypton	Gas	521–530 nm
Frequency-Doubled:YAG	Solid state	532 nm
Pulsed dye	Liquid	577–595 nm
Helium-Neon	Gas	632 nm
Ruby	Solid state	694 nm
Alexandrite	Solid state	755 nm
Diode	Solid state	800 nm
Nd:YAG	Solid state	1,064 and 1,320 nm
Diode	Solid state	1,450 nm
Erbium:Glass	Solid state	1,540 nm
Erbium:YAG	Solid state	2,940 nm
Carbon dioxide	Gas	10,600 nm

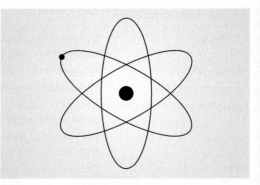

Fig. 1.1. Normal configuration of an atom with central nucleus and surrounding electrons in stable orbits

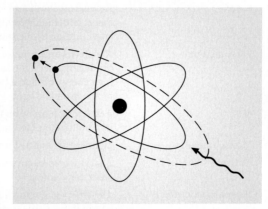

Fig. 1.2. Absorption of energy has briefly stimulated the outer electron into an unstable, but higher energy orbit.

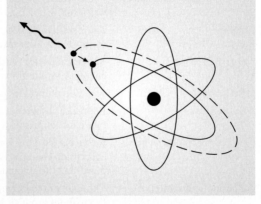

Fig. 1.3. The stimulated electron rapidly drops back to its normal orbit and assumes a stable configuration

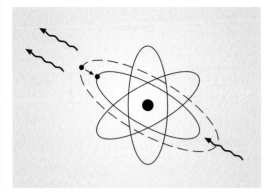

Fig. 1.4. With the stimulated emission of energy, two photons are released in phase with one another as the electron drops back to its normal, stable configuration

monochromatic or composed of a single wavelength or color. The second unique characteristic is a property known as *coherence*, where all the waves of light move together temporally and spatially as they travel together in phase with one another. The third characteristic is *collimation*, where the transmission of light occurs in parallel fashion without significant divergence, even over long distances.

■ What Is Irradiance and Energy Fluence?

In order to use a laser to treat any skin condition, it is necessary to understand how the laser can be adjusted to obtain the most desired biologic effects in tissue (Fuller 1980). Two of the factors that are important in this process are irradiance and energy fluence. *Irradiance,* also called power density, determines the ability of a laser to incise, vaporize, or coagulate tissue and is expressed in watts/cm². It can be calculated based on the formula:

$$IR = \frac{\text{laser output (watts)} \times 100}{\text{pi} \times \text{radius}^2 \text{ (of the laser beam)}}.$$

The *energy fluence* determines the amount of laser energy delivered in a single pulse and is expressed in joules/cm². It can be calculated based on the formula:

$$EF = \frac{\text{laser output (watts)} \times \text{exposure time (secs)}}{\text{pi} \times \text{radius}^2 \text{ (of the laser beam)}}.$$

In the case of irradiance and energy fluence, the higher the number the greater the effect. For example, high irradiances are needed to incise tissue, while only low irradiances are needed to coagulate tissue.

Currently Available Technology

How Does Laser Light Interact with Tissue?

In order to understand how to select the ideal laser from the myriad of currently available devices for the treatment of any cutaneous condition it is important to first understand how light produces a biologic effect in skin. The interaction of laser light with living tissue is generally a function of the wavelength of the laser system. In order for laser energy to produce any effect in skin it must first be absorbed. Absorption is the transformation of radiant energy (light) to a different form of energy (usually heat) by the specific interaction with tissue. If the light is reflected from the surface of the skin or transmitted completely through it without any absorption, then there will be no biologic effect. If the light is imprecisely absorbed by any target or chromophore in skin then the effect will also be imprecise. It is only when the light is highly absorbed by a specific component of skin that there will be a precise biologic effect. While this reaction may seem difficult to accurately anticipate, in fact, there are really only three main components of skin that absorb laser light: melanin, hemoglobin, and intracellular or extracellular water, and their absorption spectra have been well established. Manufacturers of lasers have taken this information and designed currently available technological devices that produce light which is the right color or wavelength to be precisely absorbed by one of these components of skin. This minimizes collateral injury to the surrounding normal skin.

In 1983, Drs. R. Rox Anderson and John A. Parrish (Anderson and Parrish 1983) of the Harvard Wellman Laboratories of Photomedicine published in the journal *Science* their newly developed concept of *selective photothermolysis* (SPTL). This original concept explained how to safely and effectively treat the microvessels in children with port wine stains using laser light. It also led to the first "ground up" development of a specific laser, the pulsed dye laser, to treat a specific condition–port wine stains in children. This concept has now also been used to develop more effective treatments of many other cutaneous problems including the treatment of tattoos, benign pigmented lesions, and the removal of unwanted or excessive hair. The concept of SPTL defines the way to localize thermal injury to the tissue being treated and minimize collateral thermal damage to the surrounding nontargeted tissue. This is done by choosing the proper wavelength of light that will be absorbed by the specific targeted chromophore and delivering the right amount of energy with the proper pulse duration, known as the thermal relaxation time (TRT), which is based on the physical size of the target.

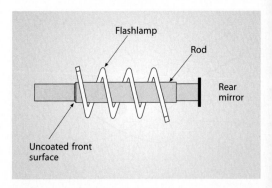

Fig. 1.5. Classic appearance of a solid state laser with central rod that could be a ruby, Nd:YAG or alexandrite crystal surrounded by a flashlamp with emission of light from only one end of the optical cavity

What Is a Q-Switched Laser?

The laser cavity "Q" is a measure of the optical loss per pass of a photon within the optical cavity (Goldman et al. 1965). Thus, the "Q" of a system is a way to characterize the quality of the photons being released so that a high "Q" implies low loss and low "Q" implies high loss. A Q-switch is a physical method to create extremely short (5–20 ns) pulses of high intensity (5–10 MW) laser light with peak power of 4 joules. In addition to the normal components (Fig. 1.5) of a laser that were previously described, this system utilizes a shutter which is constructed of a polarizer and a *pockels cell* within the optical cavity. A pockels cell is an optically transparent crystal that rotates the plane of polarization of light when voltage is applied to it. Together, the polarizer and pockels cell act as the "Q"-switch. Light energy is allowed to build (Fig. 1.6) within the optical cavity when voltage is applied to the pockels cell. Once the voltage is turned off, the light energy is released (Fig. 1.7) in one extremely powerful

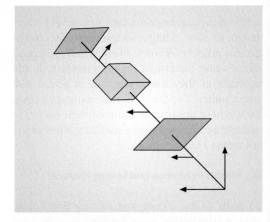

Fig. 1.6. The Q-switched lasers contain a Pockels cell that can be made opaque by the application of voltage and thus allow energy to build within the optical cavity

short pulse. Currently available Q-switched lasers include the ruby, Nd:YAG and alexandrite lasers.

The Q-switched lasers and the photons of light released from them have unique characteristics that allow them to be effectively used to treat tattoos (Goldman et al. 1967) and benign pigmented lesions. This is due to the mechanism of action whereby photoacoustic waves are generated within the skin by the released photons of light which heats the small tattoo

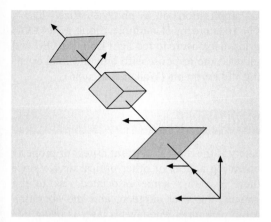

Fig. 1.7. Once the voltage is turned off, the Pockels cell becomes optically transparent and the accumulated energy is allowed to be released in a single, short, powerful pulse

pigment particles or the melanosomes. This heating causes cavitation within the cells containing the ink particles or pigment, followed by rupture and eventual phagocytosis by macrophages and removal of the debris from the site. Clinically, this process produces gradual fading of the tattoos with a series of 4–8 treatments at 6–8-week intervals and removal of the benign pigmented lesion with only 1–2 treatments, again at 6–8-week intervals. The precise targeting of subcellular organelles and pigment particles by the Q-switched lasers reduces collateral damage and minimizes the risk of scarring or textural changes. The treatment of tattoos and benign pigmented lesions represent additional examples of how selective photothermolysis can be effectively applied to more accurately treat conditions other than the microvessels of port wine stains that this concept was originally developed to treat.

Indications

Vascular Lesions

The most common laser used today for the treatment of many different vascular conditions is the pulsed dye laser (Garden and Geronemus 1990). While initially designed for the treatment

of microvessels in port wine stains of infants and children, the initial parameters have been modified to provide longer pulses and wavelengths of light to treat deeper and larger blood vessels and also to do this with epidermal cooling. Cryogen spray or contact cryogen cooling prior to the laser pulse reduces pain while also decreasing the potential for epidermal injury as the light passes through it to reach the deeper blood vessels. Thermal quenching from postpulse cooling further reduces the risk of collateral thermal injury following delivery of the pulse of light. Cooling devices are now routinely used for port wine stains in children and adults, leg veins, solar telangiectasia, and other small blood vessels diseases. Long pulses of light from the Nd:YAG laser and the nonlaser Intense Pulsed Light (IPL) devices have also been used to treat larger and deeper blood vessels. The small beam diameter of the krypton laser makes it a useful tool in the treatment of limited areas of involvement with small caliber, linear blood vessels on the nose or cheeks.

Pigmented Lesions and Tattoos

To treat cosmetically important, but benign, pigmented lesions and tattoos it is imperative that the risk of scarring and other complications be minimized as much as possible. This is made possible today with the use of short pulses of light from the Q-switched lasers, ruby, Nd:YAG, and alexandrite, that deliver pulses of light which approximate the thermal relaxation time of melanosomes and tattoo ink particles, and through their photoacoustic effects can produce destruction of melanin pigment or tattoo pigment particles for subsequent removal by macrophages. The most common benign, pigmented lesions treated with these conditions are solar lentigines, nevus of Ota/Ito, café-au-lait macules, Becker's nevus, postinflammatory hyperpigmentation, mucosal lentigines of Peutz-Jeghers syndrome, and melasma. The variability of the response in congenital or acquired nevocellular nevi makes treatment with Q-switched lasers less desirable. Decorative, traumatic, and cosmetic tattoos can all be effectively treated with the Q-switched lasers.

However, multiple treatments are required, and certain colors may not respond at all. In addition, there is a risk of darkening of some tattoo colors that occurs as a result of a chemical reaction following laser treatment, making removal exceedingly difficult.

Unwanted Hair

A number of devices, including the long-pulse ruby, long-pulse Nd:YAG, long-pulse diode, and IPL, have been used to permanently reduce the numbers of darkly pigmented hair (Wheeland 1997). This is done by targeting the melanin within the hair shaft and bulb with light energy which thermally damages the cells and either slows or destroys their ability to regrow. At present, treatment of blonde or gray hair with laser light is poor, even with the application of an exogenously applied synthetic melanin solution.

Ablative and Nonablative Facial Resurfacing

Over the past decade the short-pulsed carbon dioxide and erbium:YAG lasers have been used to perform ablative laser skin resurfacing. These devices thermally destroy the epidermis and superficial dermis with minimal collateral damage. Long healing times and even longer periods of persistent erythema and possibly permanent hypopigmentation have reduced the use of these devices. Since many patients are unwilling to accept *any* downtime from a cosmetic procedure, a number of noninvasive devices have been developed, including the Nd:YAG at 1,320 nm, the diode at 1,450 nm, the pulsed dye laser, and the IPL, to help restore the youthful condition of the skin noninvasively without producing a wound or other visible injury that would keep patients from following their normal activities. The most recent noninvasive technique for rejuvenation is using light from the light emitting diodes (LED) to stimulate the skin. This device delivers intense, non-laser, red- or blue-colored light that can stimulate fibroblasts to produce collagen, elastin, and glycosaminoglycans to help rejuvenate the skin with a series of treatments. Sometimes the topical application of a photosensitizer like a 5%–20% cream of aminolevulinic acid (ALA) prior to exposure to red light from the LED will increase the response with only minimal crusting and erythema (Walker et al. 1986).

Safety

Safety is the most important aspect of properly operating a laser or other optical device since there is always some associated risk to the patient, the laser surgeon, and the operating room personnel whenever a laser is being utilized for treatment. In the outpatient arena, the safe operation of lasers is not generally determined by the manufacturer, medical licensing board, or other regulatory body. Thus, it is important for the laser operator to understand the risks involved in using lasers and then develop an appropriate group of standards to ensure that the equipment is being used in the safest fashion possible.

Training

The safe use of any laser begins with appropriate training and familiarization in the indications and uses of each device. This allows the development of the necessary proficiency that will also result in the concomitant maximal safe use of each device.

Signage

The greatest risk when operating a laser is that of eye injury. To help prevent eye injury, appropriate signage on the laser operating room door should describe the nature of the laser being used, its wavelength, and energy. Plus, a pair of protective glasses or goggles appropriate for the device being used should always be placed on the door outside of the laser operating room in case emergency entrance is required. The door to the laser operating room should be locked, if possible, and all exterior windows closed and covered.

Eye Protection

Inside the operating room, care must also be taken to protect the eyes. If not appropriately protected, the cornea may be injured by either direct or reflected light from the carbon dioxide and erbium:YAG lasers. A more serious injury to the retina can be caused by any of the visible or near-infrared lasers. For the laser surgeon and operating room personnel there are special optically coated glasses and goggles that match the emission spectrum of the laser being used. To check whether the correct eye protection is being used the manufacturer has stamped on the arm of the glasses or the face of the goggles the wavelengths of light for which protection is provided and the amount of the protection provided in terms of optical density (O.D.). For most laser devices, the current recommendations are to use eye protection with at least an O.D. of 4.0. For the patient, there are several ways to provide appropriate eye protection. If the procedure is being performed in the immediate vicinity of the orbit, it is probably best to use metal scleral eye shields (Figs. 1.8, 1.9), which are placed directly on the corneal surface after first using anesthetic eye drops (Nelson et al. 1990). However, if the procedure is being done on the lower part of the face, trunk, or extremities, burnished stainless steel eye cups (Figs. 1.10, 1.11) that fit over the eyelids and protect the entire periorbital area are probably best.

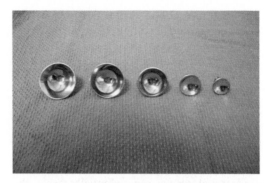

Fig. 1.9. The appearance of the convex surfaces of various sizes of corneal eye shields used to protect the eye during laser surgery in the periorbital area

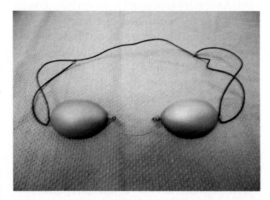

Fig. 1.10. The appearance of the Wheeland-Stefanovsky eye goggles worn over the eyelids for laser surgery not being performed in the immediate periorbital area

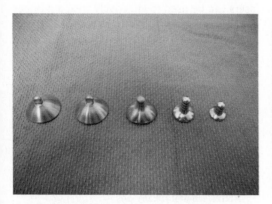

Fig. 1.8. The appearance of the concave surfaces of various sizes of corneal eye shields used to protect the eye during laser surgery in the periorbital area

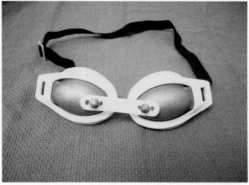

Fig. 1.11. The appearance of the externally applied Durette Oculo-Plastik eye cups worn over the eyelids during laser surgery performed closed to periorbital area

The same eye glasses or goggles used by the laser surgeon and operating room personnel are not recommended for patients since these may leave gaps on the lower edge near the cheek that permit the passage of light under them and cause injury to the patient.

Laser Plume

Any of the lasers that ablate tissue and create a plume of smoke can potentially harm the laser surgeon, patient, and operating room personnel. Various bacterial spores and human papilloma viral (HPV) particles (Garden et al. 1988) have been recovered from carbon dioxide laser plumes. The two best methods to prevent this inhalation injury are to use laser-specific surgical masks and a laser-specific plume/smoke evacuator held close to the operative site. There is no evidence that HIV or hepatitis C viral particles are transmitted in the laser plume.

Laser Splatter

When treating tattoos or benign pigmented lesions with a Q-switched laser the impact of the pulses of light can disrupt the surface of the skin, sending an explosion of blood and skin fragments flying away from the operative site at a very high speed. The speed of these particles is so fast that it cannot be removed by a smoke or plume evacuator. As a result, most the manufacturers will supply the device with a nozzle or tip that can contain these particles at the skin surface and thus prevent dissemination of these materials into the air. Another technique that has also been used successfully when treating tattoos to prevent tissue splattering from the operative site is to apply a sheet of hydrogel surgical dressing on the surface of the treatment site and discharge the laser through this material to the target. Any extrusion of tissue that occurs with the Q-switched laser pulses will be trapped within the hydrogel and not be allowed to splatter from the operative field.

Fire

Most of the medical lasers used in the treatment of skin diseases do not share the risk of older devices, like the continuous emitting carbon dioxide laser, of igniting a fire. Despite this, it is still recommended that any flammable material, including acetone cleansers, alcohol-based prep solutions, or gas anesthetics be restricted from the laser operating room. By following these simple guidelines and using common sense and skill, the risk of using a laser should be no greater than that associated with using older, traditional, nonlaser devices to perform the same procedure.

Future

As new concepts emerge to help explain how light can be used to more precisely interact with tissue, it is certain that the development of additional devices based on those concepts will follow soon after. Nonthermal *photoablative decomposition* using the femtosecond titanium:sapphire laser is but one area of recent investigation that could significantly change the way laser light can be used to ablate tissue with minimal collateral injury. Exciting new research ideas initiating photochemical reactions with laser light with either topically or parenterally administered drugs or other photosensitizers could further expand our knowledge of how lasers can be used to effectively treat a number of conditions, like inflammatory, premalignant, and malignant conditions, that currently are either poorly treated or untreatable today.

References

Anderson RR, Parrish JA (1983) Selective photothermolysis: Precise microsurgery by selective absorption of pulsed radiation. Science 220: 524–527

Arndt KA, Noe JM (1982) Lasers in dermatology. Arch Dermatol 118:293–295

Einstein A (1917) Zur Quanten Theorie der Strahlung. Phys Zeit 18:121–128

Fuller TA (1980) The physics of surgical lasers. Lasers Surg Med 1:5–14

Garden JM, O'Banion MK, Shelnitz LS, et al (1988) Papillomavirus in the vapor of carbon dioxide laser-treated verrucae. J Am Med Assoc 259: 1199–1202

Garden JM, Geronemus RG (1990) Dermatologic laser surgery. J Dermatol Surg Oncol 16:156–168

Goldman L, Blaney DJ, Kindel DJ, et al (1963) Effect of the laser beam on the skin: Preliminary report. J Invest Dermatol 40:121–122

Goldman L, Wilson RG, Hornby P, et al (1965) Radiation from a Q-switched ruby laser. J Invest Dermatol 44:69–71

Goldman L, Rockwell RJ, Meyer R, et al (1967) Laser treatment of tattoos: A preliminary survey of three years' clinical experience. J Am Med Assoc 201:841–844

Maiman T (1960) Stimulated optical radiation in ruby masers. Nature 187:493–494

Nelson CC, Pasyk KA, Dootz GL (1990) Eye shield for patients undergoing laser treatment. Am J Ophthalmol 110:39–43

Schalow AL, Townes CH (1958) Infrared and optical masers. Phys Rev 112:1940

Walker NPJ, Matthews J, Newsom SW (1986) Possible hazards from irradiation with the carbon dioxide laser. Lasers Surg Med 6:84–86

Wheeland RG (1995) Clinical uses of lasers in dermatology. Lasers Med Surg 16:2

Wheeland RG (1997) Laser-assisted hair removal Dermatol Clin 15:469

Laser Treatment of Vascular Lesions

Sean W. Lanigan

2

Core Messages

- A wide variety of cutaneous vascular disorders can be successfully treated with current lasers.
- The pulsed dye laser (PDL) enabled treatment of cutaneous vessels following principles of selective photothermolysis.
- The PDL is the most effective laser for the treatment of port wine stains but purpura limits its acceptability to patients for more cosmetic indications.
- Leg vein telangiectasia can also be treated with lasers but sclerotherapy remains the gold standard.
- Other cutaneous disorders such as psoriasis, warts, and scars can be improved by targeting the lesions' cutaneous vessels with appropriate lasers.

History

Port Wine Stain Treatment

■ Argon Laser

The earliest studies on the laser treatment of vascular disorders were on port wine stains (PWS) and published in the 1970s using both the argon and ruby lasers (Table 2.1). Most work was undertaken with the argon laser. In the 1980s this was the most frequently used laser worldwide for the treatment of PWS. The argon laser emits light at six different wavelengths in the blue green portion of the visible spectrum.

Table 2.1. Lasers used for treatment of port wine stains

Laser	Wavelength (nm)	Pulse duration (ms)
Argon	488, 514	50–200
Continuous wave dye	577, 585	50–200
Copper vapor	578	50–200
Krypton	568	50–200
Carbon dioxide (limitations see text)	10,600	50–c/w
Pulsed dye	577, 585	0.45
Long pulsed dye	585, 590, 595, 600	1.5–40
KTP	532	2–50
Alexandrite	755	3
Nd:YAG (limitations see text)	1064	50

Eighty per cent of the total emissions occur at 488 and 514 nm. These two wavelengths of light are absorbed by two chromophores in the skin: oxyhemoglobin and melanin (Fig. 2.1).

Although the argon laser wavelengths do not coincide with the absorption maxima of oxyhemoglobin, there is sufficient absorption to produce thermal damage to red blood cells in cutaneous blood vessels situated superficially within the first millimeter of the skin. Because the argon laser light is delivered in pulses lasting many tens of milliseconds (ms) there is nonspecific thermal damage to perivascular connective tissue and beyond. The unfortunate clinical consequence has been textural alteration, scarring, and pigmentary changes (Fig. 2.2)

The continuous wave argon laser beam can be mechanically shuttered to pulses of 50–

2

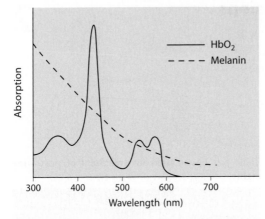

Fig. 2.1. Schematic absorption spectrum of oxyhemo-globin (Hbo₂) and melanin

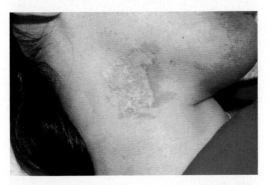

Fig. 2.2. Adverse effects of argon laser treatment [from S.W. Lanigan (2000) *Lasers in Dermatology,* Springer Verlag, London]

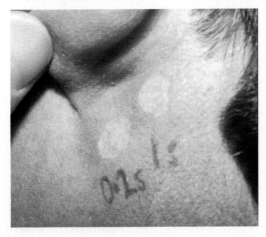

Fig. 2.3. Immediate blanching with argon laser [from S.W. Lanigan (2000) *Lasers in Dermatology,* Springer Verlag, London]

100 ms or longer. Alternatively, the operator moves the beam continuously across the surface of the skin to reduce the exposure time at each unit area. The clinical end point is minimal blanching. This is a just visible grayish white discoloration of the skin (Fig. 2.3). The operator gradually increases the power until this change is observed. The visible change of minimal blanching inevitably involves nonselective thermal damage, as it is a sign of thermal coagulation of tissue protein. Treatment is far more painful than with current lasers, and generally localized areas within a PWS are treated after infiltrational anesthesia. After treatment the skin invariably weeps and crusts with some superficial blistering. The blanched appearance reverts to a reddish purple color after a few days. Gradually after a period of 4–8 weeks the treated area visibly lightens towards normal skin color. This lightening progresses for more than 6 months after treatment. Because of the high instance of adverse reactions with the argon laser, it is essential to initially perform a small test treatment. The presence of scarring in the test site would normally indicate cessation of treatment or a change to a different laser.

Results of treating PWS with the argon laser are generally better in adults with purple PWS. Seventy per cent of adult patients will obtain good to excellent results. Hypertrophic scarring after argon laser treatment of PWS ranges from 9 to 26%. The results in children were not considered good enough and scarring rates too high to recommend the argon laser for pediatric PWS. The argon laser is rarely used now for PWS.

■ Continuous Wave Dye Laser

It was recognized early on that longer wavelengths of light absorbed by hemoglobin, particularly at 577 nm which coincides with the beta absorption peak of hemoglobin, would be more appropriate for treatment of vascular lesions (Fig. 2.1). An argon laser can be used to energize a rhodamine dye to produce coherent light at 577 or 585 nm. As with the argon laser, the light emerging is continuous but can be mechanically shuttered to produce pulses of light 10s to 100s of milliseconds in duration.

Lanigan et al. (1989) reported the results of treating one hundred patients with PWS with a continuous wave dye laser at 577 nm. A good or excellent response was seen in 63%, with a fair result in 17%; 12% of patients had a poor response. Hypertrophic scarring occurred in 5% and a similar percentage had postinflammatory hyperpigmentation. The best results were seen in older patients with purple PWS. These results were similar to those obtained with the argon laser.

Others have also found similar results with argon and continuous wave dye lasers. It is likely that any advantage gained by the longer wavelength of light is offset by the long-pulse durations employed and the use of minimal blanching as an end point. Another study evaluated 28 patients with PWS with the PDL and a continuous wave dye laser delivered through a scanning device. Results were better in 45% of patients treated with the PDL and in 15% of patients treated by the laser with scanner. There was a higher incidence of hyperpigmentation with a continuous wave laser but no differences in the instance of scarring or hypopigmentation.

■ Robotic Scanning Hand Pieces

The major disadvantage of continuous wave lasers in the treatment of PWS is the long-pulse duration resulting in nonspecific thermal damage. In addition, manual movement of a continuous wave laser beam over the skin is dependent on the operator's skill not to under- or overtreat an area. Robotic scanning devices have been developed to try and address some of these difficulties. These hand pieces can be used in conjunction with continuous wave lasers such as the argon laser, and also quasi-continuous systems, such as the copper vapor and potassium titanyl phosphate (KTP) lasers.

Robotic scanning laser devices have been most widely used in the treatment of PWS. The scanner is connected to the laser output by a fiber optic cable. The automated program places pulses of energy in a precise nonadjacent pattern in the shape of a hexagon (Fig. 2.4). The number of pulses delivered will determine the size of the hexagon, which varies from 3 to

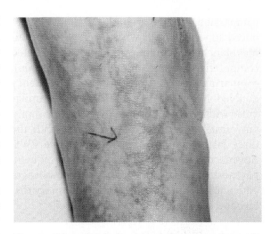

Fig. 2.4. Hexagonal clearance of a port wine stain treated with the KTP laser and robotic scanning hand piece (Hexascan) [from S.W. Lanigan (2000) *Lasers in Dermatology,* Springer Verlag, London]

13 mm in diameter. Adjacent hexagons can then be applied to cover the PWS skin. The advantages of automated scanning devices are shorter pulse durations, uniformity of energy placement, faster treatments, and reduced operator fatigue. In a study using scanning devices compared with conventional techniques the rates of scarring were substantially reduced after scanner-assisted laser treatment. Clinical results were also improved in the scanned patients.

■ Copper Vapor Laser

The copper vapor laser (CVL) is one of two heavy metal vapor lasers used clinically. Results of treating PWS with this laser were reported in the early 1990s. The wavelengths of light emitted by a CVL are 510 and 578 nm. The longer wavelength yellow light is well absorbed by oxyhemoglobin. In contrast to other yellow light lasers, the CVL emits a train of pulses with a duration of 20–25 ns and 10,000–15,000 pulses per second. Because of the very short gap between each pulse of light from the CVL, the biological effect of this laser is similar to that of a continuous wave laser. The CVL is often termed a quasi-continuous laser for this reason.

Good or excellent results have been reported in treating PWS with the CVL. Best results are seen in predominantly purple or red PWS. In comparison with the argon laser, the CVL produced superior results when used with a minimal blanching technique and a laser-associated computerized scanner. In another study (1996), comparing the CVL, argon laser, and frequency doubled Nd:YAG laser, all used with similar pulse widths and a scanner, investigators found only small differences in the results with the three lasers in the treatment of purple PWS. Adverse reactions with the CVL are infrequent, but most studies have been on small numbers of patients. Textural changes and pigmentary disturbances are most commonly reported.

■ Carbon Dioxide Laser

The use of the carbon dioxide laser for treatment of PWS is primarily of historical interest. Yet this laser may still have a role in the removal of hemangiomatous blebs within PWS which are resistant to other lasers. The carbon dioxide laser emits infrared light at 10,600 nm, which is absorbed by tissue water. In a continuous mode the laser will nonselectively vaporize tissue. It is hypothesized that if the majority of ectatic blood vessels are located superficially within the dermis, vaporization of tissue down to this level, but no further, could result in clinical lightening of the PWS without scarring. Prior to the widespread use of the PDL, the carbon dioxide laser was considered of potential value in the treatment of PWS. Lanigan and Cotterill (1990) reported their results using this laser in 51 patients with PWS. Twenty-nine of the patients had failed to respond to argon or continuous wave dye laser treatment. Twenty-two were children with pink PWS. Good or excellent results were seen in 74% of adults and 53% of children. Two children (12%) had a poor result, including a hypertrophic scar on the neck in one child. In another study the tuberous component of 30 patients with PWS was found to be unresponsive to PDL treatment. In all patients the lesions disappeared, but textural changes were seen in 37%, with one patient developing hypertrophic scarring. In view of the excellent safety profile for the PDL in the treatment of PWS, the carbon dioxide laser cannot be recommended as initial treatment of this vascular birthmark.

Currently Available Lasers for Vascular Lesions

Currently the main lasers used for the treatment of vascular lesions including PWS are PDLs and the KTP laser. Recent work has also demonstrated that long-pulsed 755-nm alexandrite and 1064-nm Nd:YAG lasers may be of value in treatment of both PWS, bulky vascular anomalies, and leg vein telangiectasia.

Indications

Lasers currently available for treating vascular disorders have a wide range of applications. Cutaneous ectatic disorders either acquired or congenital can be treated. Particular attention in this chapter will be given to the treatment of PWS, capillary (strawberry) hemangiomas, leg vein telangiectasia (Table 2.2), and facial telangiectasia. A number of other disorders of cutaneous vasculature can be treated (Table 2.3). Cutaneous disorders not primarily of vascular origin, e. g., angiolymphoid hyperplasia, adenoma sebaceum, etc., (Table 2.4) can also be treated. Particular emphasis will be given on treating psoriasis, scars, and viral warts in this way.

Table 2.2. Lasers used for treatment of leg vein telangiectasia

Laser	Wavelength (nm)	Pulse duration (ms)
KTP	532	1–200
Pulsed dye	585	0.45
Long pulsed dye	585, 590, 595, 600	0.5–40
Alexandrite	755	3–40
Diode	800, 810, 930	1–250
Nd:YAG	1064	0.3–100

Port Wine Stains

■ Port Wine Stain Treatment with the Flash Lamp Pulsed Dye Laser

The flash lamp PDL was the first laser specifically designed for the selective photo thermolysis of cutaneous blood vessels. It is considered the best laser for the overall treatment of a mixed population of patients with port wine stains (PWS), although some individuals may benefit from other lasers. The laser's active medium is a rhodamine dye selected to produce yellow light at 577–595 nm. Most lasers emit the longer wavelength as this has been shown to have a deeper depth of penetration while also retaining vascular selectivity. The pulse duration is generally fixed at 450 ms. The main variables are the spot size and fluence. The spot sizes available with today's PDL are generally between 3 and 10 mm. Five- to ten-millimeter spot sizes are generally preferred as these will cover larger areas.

Table 2.3. Other cutaneous vascular lesions treated with lasers

Spider angioma
Cherry angioma
Venous lake
Angiokeratoma
Pyogenic granuloma
Kaposi's sarcoma
Rosacea
Poikiloderma of Civatte (caution see the Sect. titled "Treatment of Other Cutaneous Vascular Lesions")
Radiation induced telangiectasia
CREST syndrome

Table 2.4. Other disorders treated by vascular specific lasers

Angiolymphoid hyperplasia
Lymphangioma
Adenoma sebaceum
Granuloma faciale
Scars
Psoriasis
Warts

There are a number of studies reporting the efficacy of the PDL in the treatment of PWS (Figs. 2.5, 2.6). Results are generally reported in terms of lightening the PWS rather than the clearance, as complete clearance only occurs in the minority of patients. The vast majority of research papers use subjective criteria for improvement compared with baseline photo-

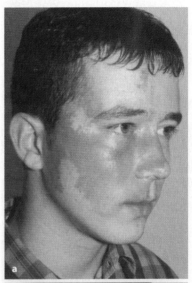

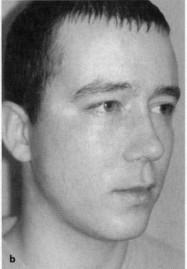

Fig. 2.5. **a** Extensive port wine stain on face (courtesy of Lasercare Clinics Ltd). **b** Near total clearance of port wine stain after course of pulsed dye laser treatment (courtesy of Lasercare Clinics Ltd)

graphy. Approximately 40% of patients with PWS achieved 75% lightening or more after laser treatment and more than 80% of PWS lightened by at least 50%. Several prognostic criteria had been put forward to assist in pre-

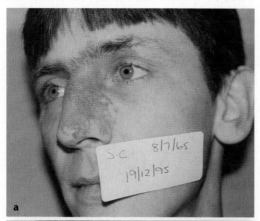

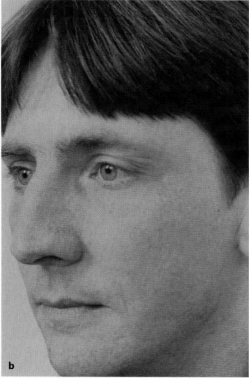

Fig. 2.6. **a** Port wine stain on face (courtesy of Laser-care Clinics Ltd). **b** Complete clearance following course of pulsed dye laser treatment (courtesy of Lasercare Clinics Ltd)

dicting the outcome of treatment. Some authors reported best results in pink lesions; others report better results in red lesions. In a study of 261 patients treated over a 5-year period (Katugampola and Lanigan 1997) color of PWS was not found to be of prognostic value. Although it is generally considered that younger children will require fewer treatments than adults, some (Alster and Wilson 1994) have reported that younger children may require more treatments owing to the rapid growth of residual blood vessels between treatments. Yet others found no evidence that treatment of PWS in early childhood was more effective than treatment at later stage.

Two features that will affect outcome are site of the PWS and size of the birthmark. PWS on the face and neck respond better than those on the leg and hand (Lanigan et al. 1996). On the face, PWS on the forehead and lateral face respond better than those over the middle of the face, particularly those involving the second branch of the trigeminal nerve. The chest, upper arm, and shoulder generally respond well. PWS less than 20 cm² at initial examination cleared more than those larger than 20 cm² irrespective of age.

■ **Second Generation Pulsed Dye Lasers**

The pulsed dye laser (PDL) has become the treatment of choice for PWS. Several investigators established the efficacy, and low incidence of side effects, of first generation PDLs operating at either 577-nm or 585-nm wavelengths and 0.45-ms pulse width. However, in the majority of cases complete clearance was not achieved, and a significant proportion of lesions were resistant to treatment. In recent years, increased understanding of the interaction between lasers and PWS has led to modification of the original PDL design and has given rise to a number of second generation lasers. The most important changes include longer pulse widths, longer wavelengths, higher delivered fluences and use of dynamic cooling devices. Many of these lasers have proven to be useful in the treatment of PWS (Geronemus et al. 2000).

Geronemus used the a 595-nm wavelength PDL, 1.5-ms pulse width and fluences up to

11–12 Jcm^{-2} with a dynamic cooling spray. They obtained greater than 75% clearing of PWS in 10 out of 16 (63%) patients after four treatments. All patients were children under 12 months of age. In another study comparing a 585-nm, 7-mm spot, 0.45-ms pulse width PDL with a second generation long-pulsed dye laser (LPDL) with 1.5-ms pulse width, 5-mm spot and wavelength settings ranging from 585 to 600 nm, optimal fading in 30 out of 62 patients was seen with the LPDL compared to only 12 patients with the shorter pulse width laser. In 20 patients there was no difference with respect to wavelength for the LPTDL; 13 patients showed best fading at 585 nm, 3 at 590 nm, 8 at 595 nm, and 6 patients at 600 nm. The authors compensated by increasing the fluence for the reduced light absorption at longer wavelengths.

In another study using a PDL with a 600-nm wavelength, superior lightening of PWS was seen in 11 out of 22 patients compared to treatment with 585 nm when compensatory fluences 1.5–2 times higher were used. At equal fluences, 585 nm produces significantly greater lightening than did the longer wavelength.

The rationale for the aforementioned alteration in treatment parameters is in part based on an increasing understanding of laser-PWS interactions from noninvasive imaging, mathematical modeling, and animal models. Longer pulse widths, as opposed to the 0.45-ms duration delivered by first generation PDLs, may be more appropriate for larger caliber PWS vessels, based on ideal thermal relaxation times of 1–10 ms (Anderson and Parish 1981; Dierickx et al. 1995). Longer wavelengths penetrate deeper, allowing targeting of deeper vessels. Higher fluences are needed in part because the newer, longer wavelength is further from the peak absorption peak of oxyhemoglobin at 577 nm (Fig. 2.1). Unfortunately, higher fluences also increase the potential for epidermal heating due to competitive absorption by epidermal melanin. This necessitates the use of cooling devices to minimize epidermal damage (and consequent side effects). Recent cooling methods include liquid cryogen sprays (Geronemus et al. 2000), cold air cooling, and contact cooling. The cooling device can be synchronized with laser pulses, or alternatively operated a few

milliseconds before or after the pulse. Studies using such epidermal cooling show a reduction in pain and prevention of pigmentary side effects during PWS treatment, even at higher fluences.

Overall, the findings of various studies indicate an improvement over the results with first generation PDLs, where greater than 75% clearing was noted in only about 40% of patients. However, with so many variables uncontrolled in the plethora of small studies, it is often difficult to clarify which modification contributed to improved outcomes.

■ Treatment of Resistant PWS

Further evidence of improved efficacy of second generation PDLs comes from responses in PWS which have proven to be resistant to first generation PDLs. In a case report, PDL treatment with a longer pulse width of 1.5 ms was effective in treating a PWS previously resistant to a 0.5-ms PDL(Bernstein 2000). Recent work using high fluence LPDL with cryogen cooling (V beam) in treatment of resistant PWS has demonstrated that further lightening can be obtained, though this may be at the expense of an increased incidence of side effects.

■ KTP Laser Treatment

The Nd:YAG laser is a solid state laser containing a crystal rod of yttrium-aluminum-garnet doped with Neodymium ions (Nd:YAG). The primary wavelength of this laser is in the infrared at 1064 nm. A frequency-doubling crystal made of KTP can be placed in the beam path to emit green light at 532 nm. This results in a quasi-continuous laser with individual pulses of 200 ns produced at a frequency of 25,000 Hz. This train of pulses can be shuttered to deliver macro pulses of 2–20 ms. High fluences are available with this laser and the pulse durations may be more appropriate for some PWS. In a preliminary investigation comparing a KTP 532 nm laser with an argon laser, 14 PWS patients were treated with both of these lasers. The results were equivalent in 12 patients and superior results were noted in 2 individuals treated with the KTP laser alone.

The KTP laser has been shown to produce further lightening in 30 PDL-resistant PWS lesions. KTP laser fluences ranged from 18 to 24 J/cm² with pulse widths of 9–14 ms. Five (17%) patients showed greater than 50% response. In general, patients preferred the KTP laser because it induced less discomfort and purpura. However, two (7%) patients developed scarring.

A study comparing the PDL with a frequency-doubled Nd:YAG laser showed similar response rates among the 43 patients; however, a substantially higher scarring rate with the 532-nm Nd:YAG laser was noted. Another study of Chinese patients showed rather modest benefits using the 532-nm Nd:YAG laser with only 13.6% of patients showing more than 50% improvement (Chan et al. 2000).

It would appear that the KTP laser has a role to play in the treatment of resistant PWS. However, the long pulses employed with this laser, and the significant epidermal injury induced by the shorter wavelength of light, may increase the incidence of laser-induced adverse effects when this laser is compared with today's PDL.

■ Infrared Lasers

Longer wavelength lasers such as the alexandrite (755 nm) and Nd:YAG (1064 nm) may have a role in PWS treatment. In the millisecond mode these lasers have been widely used for hair removal and leg vein telangiectasia. These lasers may be of value in the treatment of bulky malformations and mature PWSs. Such lesions are typically more resistant to PDL due to the predominance of larger and deeper vessels and higher content of deoxygenated hemoglobin. In one study investigators used a 3-ms alexandrite laser with dynamic cooling to treat 3 patients with hypertrophic PWS, using fluences ranging from 30 to 85 J/cm². All lesions significantly lightened without side effects. In another study 18 patients with PWS were treated, comparing a 595-nm PDL to a long-pulsed Nd:YAG laser with contact cooling. Similar clearance rates were achieved, and scarring was only noted in one patient where fluences exceeded the minimum purpura dose. Patients preferred the Nd:YAG laser because of the shorter recovery period between treatments.

■ Noncoherent Light Sources

Intense pulsed light (IPL) has also been used to treat PWS. Unlike laser systems, these nonlaser flashlamps produce noncoherent broad band light with wavelengths in the range 515 to 1200 nm and permit various pulse widths. Filters are used to remove unwanted wavelengths. The first report of thermocoagulation of PWS by polychromatic light was in 1976. In another study, a PDL-resistant PWS completely resolved after treatment with an IPL device. Another study of 37 patients treated with IPL showed a clearance of pink and red PWS, and lightening in purple PWS (Raulin et al. 1999). Direct comparison of an IPL with a PDL source in a study of 32 patients showed that overall the response rate was better with the PDL. However, it was noteworthy that 6 out of the 32 patients had a better response with the IPL. The potential role of IPL for treating PDL-resistant PWS is confirmed by a recent study showing responses in 7 out of 15 patients previously resistant to PDL, with 6 patients showing between 75% and 100% improvement (Bjerring et al. 2003). There is a multiplicity of choices of treatment parameters with noncoherent light sources. Further work is necessary to determine optimum settings.

Capillary (Strawberry) Hemangiomas

Capillary or strawberry hemangiomas are common benign tumors of infancy. Most develop during the first to the fourth week of life. There is an early proliferative phase which usually lasts for 6–9 months. This growth phase is followed by a gradual spontaneous involution which is complete in 50% by 5 years and 70% by 7 years of age.

The majority of strawberry hemangiomas are of cosmetic concern. However, the appearance of a large vascular tumor on the face of a baby is not without significance. Some hemangiomas cause problems by interference with organ function, e.g., periocular hemangiomas that lead to problems with vision. Subglottic and intranasal hemangiomas may cause problems with swallowing and respiration. Bleeding and ulceration can occur, particularly in perineal hemangiomas. Most complications occurred during the proliferative phase of the hemangiomas. Once regression is underway the majority of complications associated with the hemangioma will resolve. Unfortunately, regression of many hemangiomas is incomplete, leaving either a flat telangiectatic patch or an area of redundant discolored skin. If ulceration has occurred, scarring may follow.

Laser treatment of strawberry hemangiomas is performed either to slow or arrest proliferation in early hemangiomas, to correct or minimize complications, or cosmetically to improve residual telangiectatic lesions. Initially, the argon laser was used for the treatment of capillary hemangiomas. Treatment with this laser, however, was limited because of laser-induced textural and pigmentary changes. A continuous wave Nd:YAG laser has also been used; this laser's longer wavelength leads to deep penetration, with thermal coagulation of large volumes of tissue. It is useful for debulking large hemangiomas, but hypertrophic scarring occurs frequently. Intraoral hemangiomas can respond particularly well to this form of treatment. Lasers can also be used intralesionally in the treatment of bulky hemangiomas with both the Nd:YAG and KTP lasers. In this situation, a laser-connected fiber is inserted in the tumor and irradiation is performed as the fiber is withdrawn.

The majority of strawberry hemangiomas are currently treated with PDL. In the first report of a patient treated with PDL, a macular hemangioma was treated in a 6-day-old infant. This report and other subsequent publications emphasized the importance of *early* treatment of proliferative hemangiomas to obtain most benefit from treatment (Ashinoff et al. 1991). Because of the limited penetration depth of the PDL (just over 1 mm) it is unrealistic to expect significant alterations in a large, mature capillary hemangioma. Fluences of 5.5–6 J/cm^2 with a 5 mm spot are generally used with the 1.5 ms PDL. Treatment intervals have been reduced to every few weeks to achieve optimal benefit when treating hemangiomas. Multiple treatments may be required in small infants.

There is some controversy over the merits of early PDL treatment in uncomplicated childhood hemangiomas. In a randomized controlled study of early PDL treatment of uncomplicated childhood hemangiomas investigators have found there was no significant difference in the number of children in terms of 1-year complete clearances in the treated vs. the untreated control group. They suggested that treatment in uncomplicated hemangiomas is no better than a wait-and-see policy. This is contested by others who recommend early laser treatment especially in superficial and small childhood hemangiomas.

The deeper component of the hemangioma may still develop despite successful treatment of the superficial component. For life threatening proliferative hemangiomas, a combination of laser therapy, systemic steroids, and other agents may be required.

Of note, the complications of bleeding and ulceration respond very well to PDL therapy. Usually only one or two treatments are required and often there is a prompt response. The pain from an ulcerated hemangioma regresses noticeably and rapidly after treatment (Barlow et al. 1996). In some patients the hemangioma will also undergo regression, but this is not always the case. The entire hemangioma, not just the ulcerated or bleeding area, is generally treated.

In the incompletely regressed capillary hemangioma of the older child, superficial ectatic blood vessels can be easily treated with the PDL (Fig. 2.7), but scarring or redundant tissue may require surgical repair.

Leg Veins and Telangiectasia

Visible veins on the leg are a common cosmetic problem affecting approximately 40% of women in the United States; they remain a therapeutic challenge. Sclerotherapy is currently the gold standard of treatment, but many vessels less than 1 mm in diameter may be difficult to inject. Work over the last 5 years with vascular-specific, longer-wavelength, longer-pulsed lasers, has produced very promising results with some outcomes similar to those seen after sclerotherapy (Table 2.2).

It is important to remember in advance of laser treatment of leg vein telangiectasia to

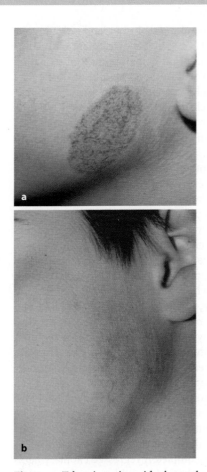

Fig. 2.7. **a** Telangiectatic residual strawberry hemangioma. **b** After pulsed dye laser treatment

examine the patient carefully to determine whether visible telangiectatic areas are secondary to venous pressure from deeper varicose veins. In the uncomplicated case, laser therapy or sclerotherapy can be considered. The majority of leg vein telangiectasia are in the range of 0.1 mm to several millimeters in diameter, much larger than the vessels in a PWS, which are 0.1 mm or less. Following the principals of selective photothermolysis, most vessels greater than 0.1 mm will require pulse durations longer than the 0.45 ms short-pulsed dye laser used for PWS. The larger the vessel, the longer the desired pulse duration. In addition, longer wavelengths of light will be required to penetrate more deeply into these deeper dermal blood vessels.

■ KTP Laser

The KTP laser produces green light at 532 nm, which is well absorbed by hemoglobin but penetrates relatively superficially. This laser does produce millisecond domain pulses, which should be appropriate for leg vein telangiectasia. However, early results with this laser in the treatment of leg veins using small spots and pulse durations of 10 ms or less were disappointing and inferior to those of the LPDL (West and Alster 1998). McMeekin (McMeekin et al. 1999) used a long-pulsed Nd:YAG laser at 532 nm to treat 10 patients with leg veins less than 1 mm in diameter. A 4 °C-chilled sapphire tip was used. One to three passes were made with fluences of 12 or 16 J/cm^2. The spot sizes were 3–5 mm in diameter. Overall, 44% of patients had more than 50% clearance following a single treatment; 94% of patients had postinflammatory hyperpigmentation, which took 6 months to clear. The required higher fluence was associated with atrophic scarring in one patient.

Others have used the same laser with a 50-ms pulse and fluences of 18–20 J/cm^2 in the treatment of 46 patients with leg veins. In patients with veins less than 1 mm in diameter, 80% had greater than 50% clearance after two treatments. In patients with veins 1–2 mm in diameter, 67% had greater than 50% clearance after two treatments. Side effects were minimal and temporary. Crusting or blistering occurred if the chill tip was not kept continuously in contact with the skin. The KTP laser seems most appropriate for superficial red telangiectasia up to 1 mm in diameter. Because there is significant absorption by melanin at 532 nm, patients with darker skin types or tanned skin will have an increased risk of side effects, including hypo- and hyperpigmentation. Contact cooling does help to reduce this side effect and allow higher fluences.

■ Long-Pulsed Dye Lasers

Based on the theory of selective photothermolysis, the predicted pulse duration ideally suited for thermal destruction of leg veins (0.1 to several millimeters in diameter) is in the 1–50-ms domain (Dierickx et al. 1995). Long PDL with wavelengths of 585–600 nm with pulse durations of 1.5 ms or longer are now available. Other investigators have treated 18 patients with leg veins ranging in diameter from 0.6 mm to 1 mm. After one treatment at 15 J/cm² 50% of vessels cleared, and at 18 J/cm² 67% of the vessels cleared. Treatments were delivered using an elliptical (2×7 mm) spot, which could be aligned over the telangiectasia. Several studies have shown this laser to be efficacious in the treatment of small vessel telangiectasia on the leg.

In another study, 80 patients with 250 leg telangiectasias were treated with the LPDL using fluences of 16–22 J/cm²; ice packs were used to cool the skin before treatment. One hundred per cent clearance was achieved in vessels with diameters up to 0.5 mm and 80% fading in vessels between 0.5 and 1.0 mm. There was no incidence of scarring, thrombophlebitis, and/or telangiectatic matting. Transient hyperpigmentation occurred in 50% of cases and hypopigmentation in 50%. Other investigators also found the 1.5-ms PDL effective in treating vessels smaller than 0.5 mm in diameter; 595 nm and 20 J/cm² with ice cube cooling were the preferred parameters. Side effects included purpura, pigmentary disturbances, and edema. Others (Weiss and Dover 2002) have also observed encouraging preliminary results using a 20-ms pulse duration 595-nm PDL.

■ **Long-Pulsed Alexandrite Laser**

There is a small peak of hemoglobin absorption in the 700–900 nm (Fig. 2.8) range of wavelengths. This has encouraged the use of longer wavelength lasers such as the alexandrite, diode, and Nd:YAG lasers in the treatment of more deeply situated, larger-caliber leg vein telangiectasia. The long-pulsed alexandrite laser emits light in the near infrared spectrum at 755 nm. The laser, when used with pulse durations of 3–20 ms theoretically penetrates 2–3 mm in depth into the skin.

Studies have evaluated the long-pulse alexandrite laser in patients with leg vein telangiectasia. By using a variety of different treatment parameters they concluded that optimal results were

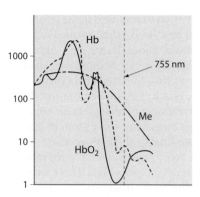

Fig. 2.8. Schematic absorption spectrum of hemoglobin (Hb), Oxyhemoglobin (Hbo2) and melanin (Me) to show absorption peak of Hb at 755 nm (courtesy of Cynosure Lasers)

achieved with 20 J/cm² and double pulses. These parameters produced almost a two-thirds reduction in vessels 0.4–1 mm in diameter after three treatments. Small vessels respond poorly if at all. Others have treated leg veins measuring 0.3–2 mm in diameter in patients with Fitzpatrick skin types I–III with a 3-ms-pulsed alexandrite laser, 8-mm spot, fluences of 60–80 J/cm², and associated dynamic epidermal cryogen cooling. Four weeks after a single treatment, 48 sites were evaluated; 35% of the treated sites had cleared by more than 75%, another 33% had cleared by more than 50%. By 12 weeks 65% of treated areas showed greater than 75% clearance. Hyperpigmentation was seen in 35% of treated areas and treatment was noted to be uncomfortable.

■ **Diode Lasers**

Diode lasers were originally introduced in the 1980s with power outputs of only 100 mW. Multiple diode laser arrays have now been developed which can be coupled directly into fiber optic delivery devices. Laser outputs have now increased to 60 W or more. Diode lasers can emit light over a broad range of wavelengths from 600 to 1020 nm. Most medical research has been with diode lasers such as gallium-arsenide (GaAs) and gallium-aluminum-arsenide (GaAlAs) emitting light in this 795- to 830-nm range.

These lasers have been used in the treatment of superficial and deep small-to-medium size leg telangiectasia. Diode lasers emit light that closely matches a tertiary hemoglobin absorption peak at 915 nm. Investigators (Varma and Lanigan 2000) have evaluated an 810-nm diode laser for the treatment of telangiectatic veins on the leg. Vessels measuring 0.5–1.5 mm in diameter were treated using fluences of 12–18 J/cm^2 with a 5-mm spot. Improvements were modest but patient acceptance was high. There were no significant side effects. Others also investigated a 940-nm diode laser in 60 patients with vessels of varying size. Best results were seen in vessels between 0.8 and 1.44 mm in diameter where 88% of patients obtained more than 75% vessel clearance. Vessels smaller than this responded poorly.

■ Long-Pulsed Nd:YAG Lasers

Several long-pulsed Nd:YAG lasers are available with pulse durations in the tens of milliseconds. These pulse widths are more appropriate in targeting large leg veins than the previous Q-switched Nd:YAG nanosecond lasers used in the treatment of tattoos. The 1064-nm infrared light is deeply penetrating with minimal absorption by melanin. When using long wavelength lasers with deeper penetration but relatively poor absorption, the combination of higher fluences and cooling devices will reduce epidermal injury.

In one study, 50 sites were evaluated with this laser. Number of pulses and fluence were altered based on vessel size. At 3-months follow-up a 75% improvement was noted. There was no epidermal injury with this laser although hyperpigmentation was common. Several studies have now demonstrated the effectiveness of the millisecond-pulsed Nd:YAG laser for lower extremity telangiectasia (Rogachefsky et al. 2002; Omura et al. 2003). Studies have focused on methemoglobin production following laser-induced heating. This methemoglobin formation leads to an increase in the absorption of the 1064-nm infrared light, adding to the effect of the Nd:YAG laser. Others (Eremia et al. 2002) compared the long-pulsed 1064-nm Nd:YAG, 810-nm diode, and 755-nm alexandrite lasers in the treatment of leg vein telangiectasia.

Vessels were 0.3–3 mm in diameter. At follow-up greater than 75% improvement was observed at 88% of the Nd:YAG laser-treated sites, 29% of the diode laser-treated sites, and 33% of the alexandrite laser-treated sites.

Despite these developments, sclerotherapy may well remain the treatment of choice for a variety of leg vein telangiectasia. A comparative study of sclerotherapy and long-pulsed Nd:YAG laser treatment (Lupton et al. 2002) showed that leg telangiectasia responded best to sclerotherapy, in fewer treatment sessions, as compared to the long-pulsed YAG laser. The incidence of adverse sequelae was equal. Laser treatment of leg vein telangiectasia appears to be of particular value in patients with telangiectatic matting and needle phobia, and for small superficial vessels too small to be treated with a needle.

Facial Telangiectasia

Facial telangiectasias are one of the commonest vascular disorders presenting for treatment. They respond readily to most lasers emitting light absorbed by hemoglobin. The two main groups of lasers used for facial telangiectasia are the pulsed dye and KTP lasers. The PDL has the lowest incidence of scarring, but may cause significant bruising after treatment (Fig. 2.9). This may not be cosmetically acceptable to patients with relatively mild disease. In a comparison of the older copper vapor laser and PDL treatment of facial telangiectasia similar improvements were seen with both lasers. However, patients preferred the linear crusting produced by the copper vapor laser compared to the purpura induced by the PDL. In a comparison study of the argon, dye, and pulsed dye lasers, the PDL was shown to produce better results. However, only 6 of 13 patients preferred this laser because of laser-induced purpura and postinflammatory hyperpigmentation. Four different frequency-doubled Nd:YAG lasers for the treatment of facial telangiectasia were assessed (Goldberg et al. 1999), using fluences of between 8 and 24/Jcm^2. The authors demonstrated equal efficacy with all such lasers and no evidence of scarring or pigmentary changes (Figs. 2.10, 2.11)

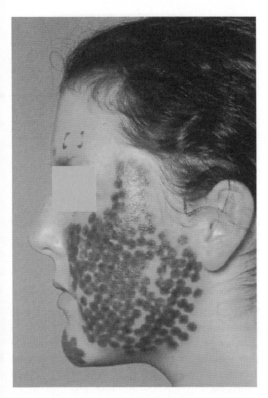

Fig. 2.9. Bruising after pulsed dye laser

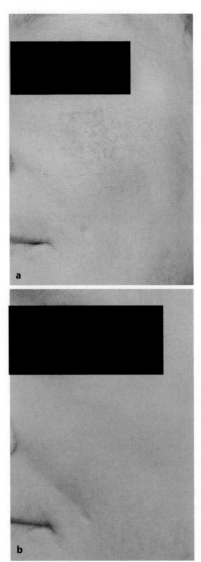

Fig. 2.10. **a** Facial telangiectasia pretreatment (courtesy of Lasercare Clinics Ltd). **b** Complete clearance after KTP laser treatment (courtesy of Lasercare Clinics Ltd)

With the development of long PDL with epidermal cooling, it may be possible to produce satisfactory improvement in facial telangiectasia while minimizing the purpura seen with the earlier PDL. Some investigators (Alam et al. 2003) have treated patients with facial telangiectasia using the PDL at fluences 1 J/cm^2 below and 0.5 J/cm^2 above the purpura threshold. There was a small reduction in observed telangiectasia with the purpura-free treatment. This was seen most commonly with finer telangiectatic vessels. A more significant reduction in telangiectasia was seen in those with laser-induced purpura. Similar work has been reported using a PDL with refrigerated air cooling and extended pulse widths of 40 ms–at fluences at or below the purpuric threshold. In all cases vessel clearance was associated with transient purpura lasting less than 7 days. The authors did not feel that it was possible, in a single treatment, to produce vessel clearance without the presence of purpura.

The addition of contact cooling when treating facial telangiectasia with the KTP laser has also been assessed. The combination of an aqueous gel with a water-cooled hand piece significantly reduced the incidence of side effects from this procedure. Yet, there was no alteration in the efficacy of clearance of telangiectasia.

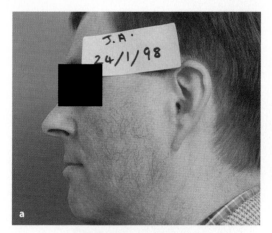 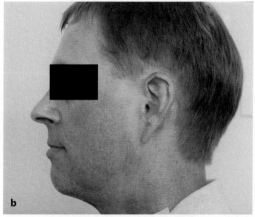

Fig. 2.11. **a** Steroid induced facial telangiectasia (courtesy of Lasercare Clinics Ltd). **b** Post-KTP laser treatment (courtesy of Lasercare Clinics Ltd)

Psoriasis

In a psoriatic plaque the capillaries of the dermal papillae are enlarged, dilated, and tortuous. A variety of lasers can be used for the treatment of psoriasis (see Chap. 6). Since the PDL can be used to treat superficial cutaneous vascular ectasias, it seemed logical to investigate whether this laser had any therapeutic efficacy in the treatment of plaque-type psoriasis. Over a decade ago there were reports of the potential benefits of the PDL in psoriasis. Subsequent studies (Katugampola et al. 1995) have confirmed the effectiveness of this treatment. Katugampola et al. treated 8 patients with chronic plaque psoriasis using the PDL at 8.5 J/cm^2 with a 5-mm spot, 3 times, over a 6-week period. Five of their 8 patients recorded an improvement of >50%, with one patient showing complete resolution. Some have performed a clinical and histological evaluation of the PDL treatment of psoriasis in 36 patients. There was no difference in response when using either a 450-µs or 1500-µs pulse duration.

Others have looked at psoriatic plaques 1 year after PDL treatment. Of nine areas completely cleared after treatment, six remained clear up to 15 months after therapy

It appears that PDL treatment can lead to improvement in psoriasis. Multiple treatments are often necessary and this technology may be inappropriate for widespread disease. Some patients with localized, resistant plaque psoriasis may benefit from this form of therapy. Further studies are required to determine the most appropriate use of this laser in the treatment of psoriasis.

Scars

PDL treatment is able to alter argon laser-induced scars, which are often erythematous and hypertrophic. By using optical profilometry measurements, researchers have shown a trend toward more normal skin texture as well as reduction in observed erythema. This work was extended to the treatment of other erythematous and hypertrophic scars using objective measurements. Investigators have noted that clinical appearance (color and height), surface texture, skin pliability, and pruritus could all be improved.

Dierickx, Goldman and Fitzpatrick (Dierickx et al. 1995; Goldman and Fitzpatrick 1995), treated 15 patients with erythematous/hypertrophic scars and obtained an average improvement of 77% after an average of 1.8 treatments. In another study 48 patients were treated with the PDL. Scars less than 1 year old responded better than those more than 1 year old. Facial scars also showed greater improvement, with an

88% average improvement with total resolution in 20% of scars after 4.4 treatments.

For persistent scars, combinations of intralesional corticosteroid injections, steroid impregnated tapes, and laser therapy may be necessary. Two studies have compared the effects of PDL treatment with other treatment modalities, particularly intralesional steroids. One study compared PDL treatment alone with laser therapy combined with intralesional corticosteroid treatment. Both treatment arms produced improvement in scars; there was no significant difference between the two treatments. Another study compared scar treatment with intralesional corticosteroids alone, combined steroids and 5-fluorouracil, 5-fluorouracil alone, or PDL treatment using fluences of 5 J/cm². All treatment areas were improved compared to baseline. The highest risk of adverse sequelae occurred in the corticosteroid intralesional group.

Other studies, however, have failed to demonstrate substantial effects of the PDL on scars. In one study, laser-treated scars were assessed using remittance spectroscopy. Although a discrete decrease in redness of the scars was reported clinically, this was not confirmed by objective data. Another prospective single blind randomized controlled study, compared laser treatment with silicon gel sheeting and controls. Although there was an overall reduction in blood volume, flow and scar pruritis over time, there were no differences detected between the treatment and control groups. Finally investigators in another study treating old and new scars with the PDL with fluences of 5–6 J/cm², were unable to demonstrate any statistical differences between treatment and control sites by photographic assessments or surface profile measurements. However, they did notice a significant improvement in scar pruritis in the laser-treated group as compared to the control group.

There are now multiple studies assessing the effects of the PDL in the treatment of scars. Although results are conflicting, particularly when controlled studies are performed, it would appear that in some cases laser therapy can be beneficial in the treatment of such scars. It is likely that vascular-induced erythema and pruritis are the two parameters that are most likely to significantly improve with this treatment.

Verrucae

Verrucae, although not truly vascular lesions, have been treated with lasers. The PDL may have potential benefits in the treatment of warts. The laser light can selectively obliterate blood vessels within the verrucae; it may also destroy the most rapidly replicating cells carrying the virus. The ability to focus the energy of the light directly on to the lesional vasculature minimizes injury to healthy skin. The PDL has been reported as successful for the treatment of resistant viral warts. In one study, 28 of 39 patients experienced resolution of the warts following an average of only 1.68 treatments with fluences of 6.5–7.5 J/cm². Warts need to be pared aggressively prior to treatment; higher fluences of 8.5–9.5 J/cm² may be necessary.

Although the PDL has been reported to be effective in the treatment of plantar warts, plantar warts appear relatively resistant to the laser treatment. In another study, 7 patients (6 plantar, 1 periungual) with recalcitrant verrucae were treated. Although there was a partial response, none of their patients experienced complete resolution of their lesions. Others treated 96 warts with only a 48% complete clearance over an average of 3.4 treatments. A study using the KTP laser at 532 nm showed complete clearing of warts in 12 of 25 patients with resistant verrucae.

There has been only one prospective randomized controlled trial comparing PDL therapy with conventional therapy in the treatment of verrucae. Forty adult patients were randomized to receive either PDL therapy (585 nm) or conventional therapy. Up to four treatments were provided at monthly intervals. One hundred and ninety four warts were evaluated. Complete response was seen in 70% of the warts treated with conventional therapy and in 66% of those in the PDL group. Thus, there was no significant difference in the treatment responses.

It should be noted that although PDL treatment is widely used in the treatment of viral warts, there are no randomized controlled studies to demonstrate the superiority of this treatment over conventional methods. While undoubtedly effective in selected patients, it is important to note that there is a significant spontaneous remission rate in viral warts. More studies with controlled trials are required.

Treatment of Other Cutaneous Vascular Lesions

Spider angiomas are easily, and successfully, treated with lasers (Table 2.3). In addition, both the pulsed dye and KTP lasers have been shown to be safe and efficacious in children. The majority of spider angiomas will clear with one or two treatments without significant complications.

Venous lakes, angiokeratomas, and cherry angiomas have all been reported to respond well to laser therapy. Tumorous outgrowths of vascular tissue such as pyogenic granulomas, nodular hemangiomas, and Kaposi's sarcoma are likely to have only a partial response owing to the limited depth of penetration of the emitted laser beam.

Areas of persistent erythema, as seen in patients with rosacea and postrhinoplasty, can be treated with the PDL (Fig. 2.12). More treatments are required than for individual telangiectasias. Purpura can be a problem when the PDL is utilized. Purpura can be diminished by using PDL-emitted longer pulse durations. In addition, the first one or two laser treatments often induces a rather spotty lightening on a background erythema, necessitating further treatment.

Matt telangiectasia seen in CREST syndrome (*c*alcinosis, *R*aynaud's phenomenon, *e*sophageal motility disorders, *s*clerodactyly, and *t*elangiectasia) can respond well to treatment (Fig. 2.13). Poikiloderma of Civatte, with its combination of pigmentation and telangiectasia seen on the lateral neck, can respond to PDL therapy. Low fluences (approximately 4 J/cm²) should be used because of the high incidence of posttreatment hypopigmentation and possible scarring seen in this disorder. Telangiectasia

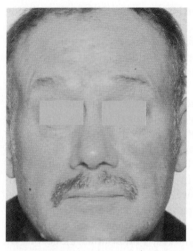

Fig. 2.12. Erythematous telangiectatic rosacea treated with pulsed dye laser (only right cheek treated)

after radiotherapy is also easily treated (Fig. 2.14).

Other lesions with a vascular component, such as angio-lymphoid hyperplasia, adenoma sebaceum, lymphangiomas (Fig. 2.15), and granuloma faciale have all been reported as successfully treated with vascular lasers. The majority of reports of these disorders have been case studies rather than controlled trials. In adenoma sebaceum, if the angio fibromas do not have a prominent vascular component, then CO_2 laser vaporization should be considered.

Disadvantages

The lasers used currently in the treatment of vascular disease have a low incidence of side effects. Risk of complications is substantially less than that seen with previously used continuous wave lasers such as the argon laser. The major disadvantage of the PDL is the development of profound purpura. Using the short-pulsed dye laser this occurred in 61 or 62 patients and lasted a mean of 10.2 days (1–21 days) (Lanigan 1995). In this same study 70% of patients reported swelling of the treated area which lasted 1–10 days; weeping and crusting occurred in 48%. Forty five per cent of patients did not go out of their home for a mean of

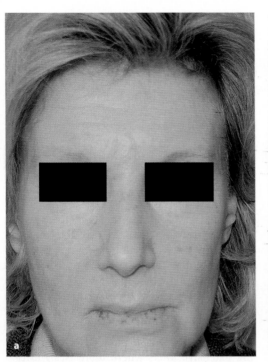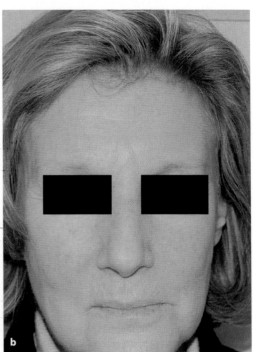

Fig. 2.13. **a** Mat telangiectasia in CREST syndrome. **b** After course of pulsed dye laser treatment

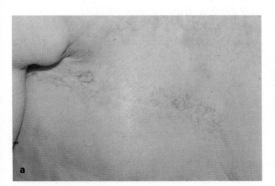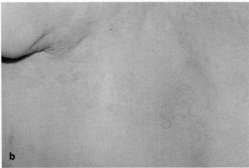

Fig. 2.14. **a** Postirradiation telangiectasia on chest wall [from S.W. Lanigan, T. Joannides (2003) Brit J Dermatol 48(1):77–79]. **b** Near total clearance after one pulsed dye laser treatment [from S.W. Lanigan, T. Joannides (2003) Brit J Dermatol 48(1):77–79]

5.6 days (2–14 days). Longer-pulsed PDL treatment leads to less purpura.

Contraindications

There are very few, if any, absolute contraindications in the use of vascular specific lasers.

There are a number of relative contraindications that the laser clinician should consider before embarking on treatment. The clinician should ascertain that the patient has realistic expectations from the laser treatment. In treating PWS, only the minority of cases will completely clear, although the majority will substantially lighten. Patients with facial telan-

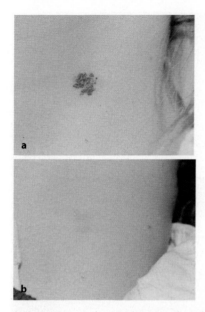

Fig. 2.15. **a** Lymphangioma on neck with prominent hemoglobin content (from S.W. Lanigan, *Lasers in Dermatology,* Springer Verlag, London 2000). **b** Good clearance of redness after pulsed dye laser treatment [from S.W. Lanigan (2000) *Lasers in Dermatology,* Springer Verlag, London]

giectasia may develop a dysmorphophobia whereby the patient is significantly disturbed by what they perceive as abnormal disfiguring changes–which are not visible to the casual observer. In general, these patients do poorly with laser treatment.

Patients who have had previous treatments to their vascular lesion, including continuous wave lasers, radiation treatment, and electrodesiccation often have some degree of scarring and hypopigmentation. This may not be obvious until the overlying vasculature has been cleared. It is important to document such changes prior to treatment. In general, patients who have had prior treatment which has resulted in scarring do not respond as well to subsequent PDL therapy.

Patients taking aspirin, nonsteroidal antiinflammatories, and anticoagulants will show more PDL-induced purpura. There have been reports of PDL-induced hypertrophic scarring in patients who have recently taken isotretinoin.

A true cause-and-effect relationship has yet to be proven.

Although laser treatment in itself is inherently safe in pregnancy, the treatment does cause pain and can be distressing. It most situations, laser may be best deferred until after delivery.

Personal Laser Technique

Facial Telangiectasia

It is extremely important when assessing patients for treatment of their facial telangiectasia that they are made fully aware of the available procedures and the likely outcomes and side effects (Fig. 2.16). In general, patients with small, fine, relatively superficial telangiectasia can be treated with most available lasers. Most patients will prefer the KTP laser because of the reduced associated purpura. Also, when treating extensive areas where there is significant background erythema, the PDL is likely to produce a superior result. Generally, I perform a test patch in this group of patients.

When using the PDL, although it may be possible to clear the problem without purpura, it is my experience that such an approach generally requires multiple treatments. I attempt to produce vessel damage with fluences as close to the purpura threshold as possible. Most patients do not require local anesthesia for this procedure. A disadvantage of topical anesthetics is the vasoconstriction that occurs, which may make it difficult to see all the vessels. The combination of concurrent epidermal cooling and longer pulse durations will reduce the PDL-induced purpura. Patients should avoid traumatizing the area after treatment and use potent sunscreens. Treatments are generally repeated at 4- to 6-week intervals until vessel clearance has occurred. In general, most patients need between two and four treatments.

When using the KTP laser, the object is to heat seal the vessels under direct observation. This treatment requires more skill and training than when using the PDL. The target vessel is traced with the laser beam using relatively small spot sizes and repetition rates of 3–8 Hz. This

AGREEMENT/CONSENT FOR VASCULAR LASER TREATMENT

This agreement is between . . . . Clinics and Doctor/Nurse . . . .

and (Mr, Mrs, Miss, Ms) . . . .
(Full name of patient) hereafter known as the patient.

1. Please read this form and the notes very carefully.
2. If there is anything you do not understand about the explanation, or if you want more information, please ask the clinician.
3. Please check that all the information on the form is correct. If it is, and you feel happy with all the explanations given please sign the form.

I the patient understand:
1. The efficacy of the treatment with lasers varies from individual to individual and I understand that a small percentage of patients may fail to respond to treatment and I as an individual may not respond.
2. The treatment that I receive will be appropriate for my specific needs and will be given by an appropriately trained member of the clinic.
3. I understand I must give staff all the relevant medical details prior to treatment.
4. A test patch may be necessary before commencing treatment with lasers.
5. Following treatment the skin will be red, and if the Pulsed Dye laser has been used there will be bruising. Swelling, blistering or crusting can occur and may take several days to resolve, the bruising will take longer (as with any normal bruise).
6. Following treatment I will be given an aftercare sheet, which I should follow. Treated areas should not be picked, scratched or traumatized and should be kept well moisturized.
7. Following treatment there may be hypopigmentation or hyperpigmentation (marked lightening or darkening of the skin). While these reactions are not common there is a possibility that they can occur. However, in time, these will usually fade away, although hypopigmentation may be permanent, I have been advised to use a total sunblock cream. I understand that following my course of treatment I must wear sunblock for a minimum of six weeks to avoid possible postinflammatory hyperpigmentation.
8. There is a 1%–5% risk of scarring with laser treatment of this kind.
9. I understand that photographs will be taken before and during my treatment and that these photographs remain the property of the clinic although I may have access to them at any time.
10. **I understand that it is my responsibility prior to each treatment undertaken that I inform the doctor or nurse of any changes in medical status, including medication or herbal remedies I am taking.**
11. I understand that if I have a suntan I may not be offered treatment; during treatment I have been advised not to use sunbeds.

The patient acknowledges that he/she has read and fully understood this agreement before signing it and has also read and understood any information sheets that they have been given.

I understand and agree to .... terms of business and understand that I can request an additional copy of these terms at any time.

Patient's signature . . . .

Fig. 2.16. Consent form

procedure is made easier using illuminated magnification. The aim is to see disappearance of the vessel without obvious epidermal changes, particularly white lines. A few small test areas are performed altering the fluence, pulse width, or repetition rate to achieve this. Starting parameters could be 6–12 J/cm^2, 3–6 ms with a 1- or 2-mm beam diameter. It may be helpful to use concurrent cooling during the procedure. Immediately afterwards the patients will experience quite marked reactive erythema. This can be reduced with cool dressings and topical aloe vera. The erythema usually clears within 24 hours, but some crusting may occur. Large areas of crusting, blistering, or erosion suggest that treatment has been too aggressive.

Port Wine Stains

Pretreatment assessment of the patient should include a record of previous treatment and its effects. Argon laser treatment in particular can produce frequent pigmentary disturbances, especially hypopigmentation, which may not be obvious in a partially treated PWS. It will become very obvious after successful PDL therapy. Scarring from previous treatment should be recorded. The patient should be advised not to expose their skin to sunlight, as a tan overlying the PWS will interfere with therapy. Good quality, standardized color photographs should be taken at baseline and throughout the treatment course. It is useful to show the patients a portfolio of photographs to illustrate the procedure, in particular the bruising that will occur after treatment.

The fluence to be used can be determined by performing a test treatment over a range of fluences and reviewing the patients 6–8 weeks later. The lowest fluence producing lightening of the PWS can be used. As a general rule, with a 7-mm spot, fluences are in the range of 4.5–8 J/cm^2. The lower range of fluences should be used in both the pediatric patient and more sensitive anatomic areas. As treatment progresses with lightening of the PWS, it is reasonable to cautiously increase the fluence by 0.25–0.5 J/cm^2 to maintain improvement. It has been shown, however, that not all PWS will clear

with PDL treatment. Repeatedly increasing the fluence in the nonresponding PWS will unfortunately increase the likelihood of an adverse reaction, such as scarring.

PDL treatment causes discomfort or pain to the patient described as a sharp stinging sensation similar to being flicked with an elastic band. This stinging is replaced immediately by a hot pruritic sensation. Some individuals appear to be able to tolerate large treatments without distress, but this should not be assumed. Two percent of patients surveyed described severe pain after treatment despite attempts at adequate analgesia (Lanigan 1995).

Topical anesthetic agents can assist patients. A eutectic mixture of local anesthetic (EMLA) cream containing lidocaine 2.5% and prilocaine 2.5% has been shown effective in reducing PDL-induced pain (Lanigan and Cotterill 1989). The cream must be applied thickly under occlusion to the PWS for 90 min to 4 h before treatment. It is not indicated for children under 1 year. An alternative to EMLA is Ametop, a 4% amethocaine gel which has the advantage of a more rapid onset of action of 30–45 min. It also should be applied under occlusion and is not recommended in infants under 1 month. There are concerns of excessive absorption of Ametop on highly vascular surfaces. Large areas should not be treated with this drug. Skin irritation and allergic rashes can occur from these creams. Despite correct techniques, sensitive areas of the face, especially the upper lip and periorbital areas, may not be adequately anesthetized with topical creams. Additional infiltrational and nerve block anesthesia can be used to supplement the topical agents; unfortunately this in itself can be traumatic for the patient.

In children these topical anesthetic techniques are often not enough. In my experience the majority will require general anesthesia. Some authors advocate sedation in combination with other anesthetic techniques without general anesthesia. The procedure can cause anxiety in children as well as discomfort, as their eyes are covered while the laser emits noises as well as light during the treatment. After the test treatment, each further laser procedure involves placement of laser impacts over the whole PWS using the lowest fluence to achieve lightening.

This needs to be reduced over the eyelids, upper lip, and neck. Each impact of the laser produces a visible purpuric discoloration, which appears either immediately or within minutes. This is a sharply demarcated circle, which allows the operator to place the next spot adjacent to it. For PDL with gaussian beam profiles, spots should be overlapped by approximately 10%. This will reduce the tendency in some patients to a spotty appearance as the PWS clears. Other PDLs may have different beam profiles and a decision on whether to overlap spots can only be made on the basis of knowledge of the beam energy profile.

After treatment of the PWS, most patients will note purpura for 7–14 days. A minority will have purpura up to 28 days. Small areas may crust or weep, but large areas of blistering suggest reduction of the fluence at the next treatment. The greatest reaction after treatment occurs early in the course of therapy or after increasing the fluence. After each treatment the PWS should be lighter in appearance. Treatments are repeated at an interval of about 8 weeks. Gradually through a course of treatment the lightening after each treatment gets less until no further progress between visits can be seen. The majority of patients who experienced satisfactory lightening of their PWS do so in their first four to ten treatments. Although improvements can occur beyond 20 treatments, the small benefits should be balanced against the morbidity produced by treatment (Kauvar and Geronemus 1995).

Postoperative Care

There is minimal postoperative care required after treatment with today's vascular lasers. In most cases the epidermis will be intact, but in a significant minority there will be some blistering. The first consideration after treatment is to deal with discomfort. This pain can be lessened by cooling the skin either with refrigerated air blowing, cold compresses, spraying with water, or aloe vera. With the PDL this cooling can be repeated until pain and discomfort has eased. The area can then be kept moisturized with an emollient. If treatment has been performed close to or around the eye there will be a risk of periocular edema. Patients should be instructed to sleep with an extra pillow to encourage gravitational removal of leaked edema fluid. The area can be washed gently with soap and water. No make-up can be applied until after any crusting has settled.

With the KTP laser and other continuous wave lasers there may be some blistering and crusting. The operator may consider use of topical antibiotics. There is little evidence to suggest this is required. Patients can also be instructed to take analgesia as needed. All patients should be instructed on the absolute importance of not picking or scratching at treated areas. They will also need to use a total sunblock preparation to lessen postinflammatory hyperpigmentation. Inability to comply with this will significantly reduce the effectiveness of the procedure.

Complications

All persistent side effects are generally due to pigmentary changes and/or scarring. Postinflammatory hyperpigmentation is the commonest side effect and has been reported to occur between 10% and 27% of the time in treated patients. Hyperpigmentation is most common in treated PWS on the leg and is reversible. Hypopigmentation occurs in up to 2.6% of patients and generally occupies only a small area of the treated lesion. Atrophic scarring occurs in 1%–5%; hypertrophic scarring in less than 1% of PDL-treated patients. Atrophic textural changes often improve spontaneously over 6–12 months.

Rarer side effects occasionally reported include atrophie blanche-like scarring, dermatitis, and keloid formation during Isotretinoin therapy. A case has been reported of leg ulceration after PDL treatment of a vascular malformation.

Even when using long PDL to lessen purpura, significant facial edema can develop. Alam (Alam et al. 2003) reported postoperative edema in 87% of 15 patients with purpuric-free laser parameters. This included 27% of patients with symptomatic eye swelling.

The KTP laser, which has longer pulse durations and a wavelength which is also absorbed by melanin, has a higher incidence of mild side effects due to epidermal injury. These may be pain, redness, vesiculation, and crusting. These side effects are transient, and in the treatment of facial telangiectasia are not generally associated with long-term problems. There is a risk of atrophic scarring with this laser. This will occur more commonly when treating paranasal areas, as these vessels frequently require more aggressive treatment parameters. Concurrent epidermal cooling will significantly reduce the incidence of side effects after treatment with this laser.

The Future

Significant advances have been made in recent years in the technological development of lasers that can target cutaneous vascular disorders by selective photothermolysis. However, results in PWS in particular can still be disappointing.

A number of investigators are pursuing a greater understanding of the vascular responses of PWS to lasers through noninvasive imaging and mathematical modeling. The eventual goal is to tailor laser therapy to individual PWS characteristics by altering both laser type and parameter settings. For example, some have designed a photoacoustic probe which allows in vivo determination of PWS depth. Others have demonstrated that videomicroscopy can be used to assess treatment response in relation to vessel depth. Still others have used optical Doppler tomography to perform real-time imaging of blood flow within PWS. Partial restoration of blood flow occurring immediately or shortly after laser exposure was indicative of reperfusion due to inadequate vessel injury. By using this imaging method, they proposed that PWS could be retreated with higher fluences in a step-wise manner, until a permanent reduction in blood flow occurs. This would be indicative of irreversible vessel damage and expected clinical lightening.

Despite the recent advances made, it remains difficult to fully eradicate PWS with our current armamentarium of lasers and non-coherent light sources. Alternative therapies including photodynamic therapy are being considered. The considerable work in this field reinforces the notion that PWS display considerable clinical and histological heterogeneity. This is likely to mean that a number of approaches will be needed to optimize treatment of PWS. There is a clear need for further trials, particularly to establish the role of noncoherent light sources and lasers, other than the PDL. To ensure comparability of future studies, common objective clinical outcome measures need to be employed, together with, where possible, noninvasive imaging techniques which can increase our understanding of laser-PWS interactions. However, we should also recognize the importance of incorporating measures of patient satisfaction into study design, since after all, it is patients' own assessments which ultimately reflect treatment outcomes.

References

Alam M, Dover JS, Arndt KA (2003) Treatment of facial telangiectasia with variable-pulse high-fluence pulsed-dye laser: comparison of efficacy with fluences immediately above and below the purpura threshold. Dermatol Surg 29(7):681–684

Alster TS, Wilson F (1994) Treatment of port-wine stains with the flashlamp-pumped PDL: extended clinical experience in children and adults. Ann Plast Surg 32(5):478–484

Anderson RR, Parish JA (1981) Microvasculature can be selectively damaged using dye lasers: a basic theory and experimental evidence in human skin. Lasers Surg Med 1:263–276

Ashinoff R, Geronemus RG (1991) Capillary hemangiomas and treatment with the flash lamp-pumped pulsed dye laser. Arch Dermatol 127(2):202–205

Barlow RJ, Walker NP, Markey AC (1996) Treatment of proliferative hemangiomas with the 585 nm pulsed dye laser. Br J Dermatol 134(4):700–704

Batta K, Goodyear HM, Moss C, Williams HC, Hiller L, Waters R (2002) Randomized controlled study of early pulsed dye laser treatment of uncomplicated childhood hemangiomas: results of a 1-year analysis. Lancet 360(9332):521–527

Bernstein EF (2000) Treatment of a resistant port-wine stain with the 1.5-msec pulse duration, tunable, pulsed dye laser. Dermatol Surg 26(11):1007–1009

Bjerring P, Christiansen K, Troilius A (2003) Intense pulsed light source for the treatment of dye laser resistant port-wine stains. J Cosmet Laser Ther 5:7–13

Chan HH, Chan E, Kono T, Ying SY, Wai-Sun H (2000) The use of variable pulse width frequency doubled Nd:YAG 532 nm laser in the treatment of port-wine stain in Chinese patients. Dermatol Surg 26(7): 657–661

Dierickx CC, Casparian JM, Venugopalan V, Farinelli WA, Anderson RR (1995) Thermal relaxation of port wine stain vessels probed in vivo: the need for 1–10 millisecond laser pulse treatment. J Invest Dermatol 105:709–714

Eremia S, Li C, Umar SH (2002) A side-by-side comparative study of 1064 nm Nd:YAG, 810 nm diode and 755 nm alexandrite lasers for treatment of 0.3–3 mm leg veins. Dermatol Surg 28(3):224–230

Fitzpatrick RE, Lowe NJ, Goldman MP, Borden H, Behr KL, Ruiz-Esparza J (1994) Flashlamp-pumped pulsed dye laser treatment of port-wine stains. J Dermatol Surg Oncol 20(11):743–748

Geronemus RG, Quintana AT, Lou WW, Kauvar AN (2000) High-fluence modified pulsed dye laser photocoagulation with dynamic cooling of port wine stains in infancy. Arch Dermatol 136:942–943

Goldberg DJ, Meine JG (1999) A comparison of four frequency-doubled Nd:YAG (532 nm) laser systems for treatment of facial telangiectases. Dermatol Surg 25(6):463–467

Katugampola GA, Lanigan SW (1997) Five years' experience of treating port wine stains with the flashlamp-pumped pulsed dye laser. Br J Dermatol 137:750–754

Kauvar AN, Geronemus RG (1995) Repetitive pulsed dye laser treatments improve persistent port-wine stains. Dermatol Surg 21(6):515–521

Lanigan SW (1996) Port wine stains on the lower limb: response to pulsed dye laser therapy. Clin Exp Dermatol 21(2):88–92

Lanigan SW, Cartwright P, Cotterill JA (1989) Continuous wave dye laser therapy of port wine stains. Br J Dermatol 121(3):345–352

Lupton JR, Alster TS, Romero P (2002) Clinical comparison of sclerotherapy versus long-pulsed Nd:YAG laser treatment for lower extremity telangiectasias. Dermatol Surg 28(8):694–697

McMeekin TO (1999) Treatment of spider veins of the leg using a long-pulsed Nd:YAG laser (Versapulse) at 532 nm. J Cutan Laser Ther 1(3):179–180

Omura NE, Dover JS, Arndt KA, Kauvar AN (2003) Treatment of reticular leg veins with a 1064 nm long-pulsed Nd:YAG laser. J Am Acad Dermatol 48(1): 76–81

Raulin C, Schroeter CA, Weiss RA, Keiner M, Werner S (1999) Treatment of port wine stains with a noncoherent pulsed light source: a retrospective study. Arch Dermatol 135:679–683

Rogachefsky AS, Silapunt S, Goldberg DJ (2002) Nd:YAG laser (1064 nm) irradiation for lower extremity telangiectasias and small reticular veins: efficacy as measured by vessel color and size. Dermatol Surg 28(3):220–223

Varma S, Lanigan SW (2000) Laser therapy of telangiectatic leg veins: clinical evaluation of the 810 nm diode laser. Clin Exp Dermatol 25(5):419–422

Weiss RA, Dover JS (2002) Laser surgery of leg veins. Dermatol Clin 20(1):19–36

West TB, Alster TS (1998) Comparison of the long-pulse dye (590–595 nm) and KTP (532 nm) lasers in the treatment of facial and leg telangiectasias. Dermatol Surg 24(2):221–226

Laser Treatment of Pigmented Lesions

CHRISTINE C. DIERICKX

Core Messages

- Accurate diagnosis of pigmented lesions is mandatory before laser treatment.
- For some pigmented lesions, laser treatment may be the only treatment option.
- Tattoos respond well to Q-switched lasers.
- Amateur and traumatic tattoos respond more readily to treatment than do professional tattoos.
- Cosmetic tattoos should be approached with caution.
- Treatment of melanocytic nevi remains controversial, but worth pursuing.

History

Selective Photothermolysis

The idea of treating cutaneous pigmented lesions with lasers was first tested in the early 1960s with the use of a normal mode ruby laser. This research indicated that the target was the melanosome. Unfortunately, due to laboratory difficulties, further research was halted.

In the past 15 years selective photothermolysis has largely transformed dermatologic laser surgery. The term *selective photothermolysis* describes site-specific, thermally mediated injury of microscopic tissue targets by selectively absorbed pulses of radiation (Anderson 1983). Three basic elements are necessary to achieve selective photothermolysis: (1) a wavelength that reaches and is preferentially absorbed by the desired target structures, (2) an exposure duration less than or equal to the time necessary for cooling of the target structures, and (3) sufficient fluence to reach a damaging temperature in the targets. When these criteria are met, selective injury occurs in thousands of microscopic targets, without the need to aim the laser at each one.

At wavelengths that are preferentially absorbed by chromophoric structures such as melanin-containing cells or tattoo-ink particles, heat is created in these targets. As soon as heat is created, however, it begins to dissipate by conduction. The most selective target heating is achieved when the energy is deposited at a rate faster than the rate for cooling of the target structures. In contrast to diffuse coagulation injury, selective photothermolysis can achieve high temperatures in structures or individual cells with little risk of scarring because gross dermal heating is minimized.

Pigmented Lesion Removal by Selective Photothermolysis

Because melanin absorbs light at a wide range of wavelengths – from 250 to 1200 nm – several lasers or intense pulsed light sources can effectively treat pigmented lesions. For tattoos, light absorption depends on the ink color, but the predominant color (blue-black) also absorbs well throughout the 532–1064-nm range. Almost any laser with sufficient power can be used to remove benign pigmented lesions of the epidermis. The selective rupture of skin melanosomes was first noted by electron microscopy in 1983, after 351-nm, submicrosecond excimer laser pulses of only about 1 J/cm^2. At fluences damaging melanocytes and pigmented keratinocytes, epidermal Langerhans cells apparently escape injury.

With regard to wavelength, absorption by melanin extends from the deep UV through visible and well into the near-IR spectrum. Across this broad spectrum, optical penetration into skin increases from several micrometers to several millimeters. One would therefore expect melanosomes and the pigmented cells containing them to be affected at different depths across this broad spectrum.

A variety of thermally mediated damage mechanisms are possible in selective photothermolysis, including thermal denaturation, mechanical damage from rapid thermal expansion or phase changes (cavitation), and pyrolysis (changes in primary chemical structure). Mechanical damage plays an important role in selective photothermolysis with high-energy, submicrosecond lasers for tattoo and pigmented lesion removal. The rate of local heating and rapid material expansion can be so severe that structures are torn apart by shock waves, cavitation, or rapid thermal expansion.

Grossly, the immediate effect of submicrosecond near-UV, visible, or near-IR laser pulses in pigmented skin is immediate whitening. This response correlates very well with the melanosome rupture seen by electron microscopy and is therefore presumably a direct consequence of melanosome rupture. A nearly identical but deeper whitening occurs with Q-switched laser exposure of tattoos, which like melanosomes consist of insoluble, submicrometer intracellular pigments. Although the exact cause of immediate whitening is unknown, it is almost certainly related to the formation of gas bubbles that intensely scatter light. Over several to tens of minutes, these bubbles dissolve, causing the skin color to return to normal or nearly normal. In addition, pyrolysis may occur at the extreme temperatures reached within melanosomes or tattoo ink particles, directly releasing gases locally. Regardless of its cause, immediate whitening offers a clinically useful immediate endpoint that apparently relates directly to melanosome or tattoo ink rupture (Fig. 3.1).

Melanin in both the epidermis (as in cafe-au-lait macules and lentigines) and the dermis (as in nevus of Ota), as well as dermal tattoo particles, is an important target chromophore for laser selective photothermolysis. Clinically,

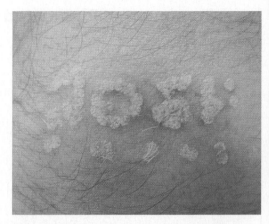

Fig. 3.1. Immediate whitening after laser treatment

selective photothermolysis is highly useful for epidermal and dermal lesions in which cellular pigmentation itself is a cause. These include lentigines, cafe-au-lait macules (which display a high rate of recurrence), nevus spilus, Becker nevi, blue nevi, and nevus of Ota. However, selective thermolysis has only been variably effective for dermal melasma, postinflammatory hyperpigmentation, or drug-induced hyperpigmentation.

Currently Available Technology

Lasers and Intense Pulsed Light Sources Used to Treat Pigmented Lesions and Tattoos

■ **Continuous-Wave Lasers (CW Lasers)**

Although Q-switched lasers are now the modality of choice for most pigmented lesions, continuous-wave and quasi-continuous lasers, when used properly, can also be effective (Tables 3.1, 3.2, 3.3). The lasers include the CW argon laser (488 and 514 nm), a CW dye laser (577 and 585 nm), a CW krypton (521–530 nm), a quasi-CW copper vapor laser (510 and 578 nm), an erbium (2940 nm) and CO_2 (10,600 nm) laser.

The CW and quasi-CW visible light lasers can be used to selectively remove pigmented lesions. However, because of the shorter wavelengths of these lasers, they penetrate only superficially. Thus, they are effective only for

Table 3.1. Long pulse lasers for treatment of pigmented lesions

Light source	Wavelength (nm)	System name	Pulse duration (ms)	Fluence (J/cm²)	Spot size (mm)	Repetition rate (Hz)	Other features
Long pulse ruby	694	E2000 (Palomar)	3, 100	10–40	10, 20	1	Cooling handpiece 0–100°C; Fiber delivery; Photon recycling
		Epitouch Ruby (Sharplan)	1.2	10–40	3–6	1.2	Triple pulse technology
		Ruby Star (Aesclepion-Meditec)	4	Up to 35	Up to 14	1	Dual mode: may also be Q-switched
		Sinon (Wavelight)	4	Up to 30	5, 7, 9	0.5–2	Cold air unit; May also be Q-switched
Long pulse alexandrite	755	Apogee (Cynosure)	0.5–300	25–50	5, 10, 12, 15	3	Cold air or integrated cooling
		Gentlelase (Candela)	3	10–100	6, 8, 10, 12, 15, 18	Up to 1.5	Dynamic cooling device
		Epitouch ALEX (Sharplan)	2–40	Up to 50	5, 7, 10	1	Scanner option
		Ultrawave II/III (Adept Medical)	5–50	5–55	8, 10, 12	1–2	Available with 532-nm and/or 1064-nm Nd:YAG
		Epicare (Light Age)	3–300	25–40	7, 9, 12, 15	1–3	
		Arion (WaveLight)	1–50	Up to 40	6, 8, 10, 12, 14	Up to 5	Cold air unit
Diode laser	800	LightSheer (Lumenis)	5–400	10–100	9×9, 12×12	Up to 2	Cooling handpiece
		Apex-800 (Iridex)	5–100	5–60 (600 W)	7, 9, 11	Up to 4	Cooling handpiece
		SLP1000™ (Palomar)	5–1000	Up to 575	12	Up to 3	SheerCool triple contact cooling, photon recycling
		MedioStar (Aesclepion-Meditec)	50	Up to 64	10, 12, 14	Up to 4	

3

Table 3.1. Long pulse lasers for treatment of pigmented lesions (continued)

Light source	Wavelength (nm)	System name	Pulse duration (ms)	Fluence (J/cm²)	Spot size (mm)	Repetition rate (Hz)	Other features
Diode laser		F1 Diode Laser (Opusmed)	15–40	10–40	5, 7	4	
Long pulse Nd:YAG	1064	CoolGlide (Cutera)	0.1–300	up to 300	3, 5, 7, 10	Up to 2	Contact precooling
		Lyra (Laserscope)	20–100	5–900	10		Contact cooling Photon recycling
		Ultrawave I/II/III (Adept Medical)	5–100	5–500	2, 4, 6, 8, 10, 12	1–2	Available with 532-nm Nd:YAG and/or 755-nm alexandrite
		Gentle Yag (Candela)	0,25–300	Up to 600	1,5, 3, 6, 8, 10, 12, 15, 18optional	Up to 10	Cryogen spray
		VARIA (CoolTouch)	300–500	Up to 500	3–10		Pulsed cryogen cooling with Thermal Quenching
		Acclaim 7000 (Cynosure)	0,4–300	300	3, 5, 7, 10, 12	5	Cold air or integrated cooling
		Smartepil II (Cynosure)	Up to 100	16–200	2,5, 4, 5, 7, 10	6	Smart cool Scanner
		Dualis (Fotona)	5–200	Up to 600	2–10		
		Vasculight Elite (Lumenis)	2–16	70–150	6	0.33	Combined with IPL
		Profile (Sciton)	0,1–200	Up to 400			
		Mydon (WaveLight)	5–90	10–450	1,5, 3, 5, 7, 10	1–10	Contact or air cooling

Table 3.2. Q-Switched lasers for treatment of pigmented lesions and tattoos

Light source	Wavelength (nm)	System name	Pulse duration (ns)	Fluence (J/cm²)	Spot size (mm)	Repetition rate (Hz)	Other features
Q-switched ruby	694	Sinon (Wavelight)	20	Up to 15	3, 4, 5	0,5–2	Cold air unit (optional) Also long pulse
		Spectrum RD-1200 (Palomar)	28	3–10	5, 6, 5	0,8	
		Ruby Star (Aesclepion-Meditec)	30	Up to 10	Up to 5	1	Dual mode: may also be Q-switched
Q-switched Alexandrite	755	Accolade (Cynosure)	60	7–30	2.4, 3, 5	Up to 5	
		Ta2 Eraser (Light Age)	60	7.5	4	8–10	
		Alexlazr (Candela)	50	Up to 12	2, 3, 4	Up to 5	
Q-switched Nd:YAG	532/1064	Softlight (Thermolase)	12–18	2.5–3	7	Up to 10	Only 1064 nm
		MedLite C6 (HOYA/ConBio)	<20	Up to 12	3, 4, 6, 8	Up to 10	532 and 1064 nm
		Q-Clear (Light Age)		2–12	2, 3, 4	1–6	532 and 1064 nm
		Q-YAG 5 (Palomar)	3	Up to 12,5	2, 4, 6	Up to 10	532 and 1064 nm

3

Table 3.3. Intense pulsed light sources treatment of pigmented lesions

Light source	System name	Spectrum (nm)	Optical filter for pigment (nm)	Pulse duration (ms)	Pulse delay (ms)	Fluence (J/cm²)	Spot size (mm)	Special features
IPL	Ellipse Flex (DDD, Horsholm Denmark)	400–950	555–950	2 × 2.5	10	8–10	10 × 48	Dual mode filtering technique
IPL	Quantum SR (Lumenis)	560–1200		6–2	5–60	15–45	8 × 34	
IPL	Prolite (Alderm, Irvine, CA)	550–900	550–900	2	2	10–50	10 × 20 20 × 25	FLP (fluorescent pulsed light)
IPL	Photolight (Cynosure Chelmsford, MA)	400–1200	550–1200	5–50		3–16	46 × 18	Xenon pulsed lamp
IPL	Quadra Q4 (Derma Med USA)	510–1200		48		10–20	33 × 15	Quad pulsed light system
IPL	Skinstation (Radiancy Orangeburg, NY°)	400–1200		35		4–7	35 × 12	Light heat energy (LHE)
IPL	Spectrapulse (Primary Technology, Tampa, FL)	510–1200		3 × 12	4 and 5 Resp	10–20	15 × 33	Light energy recycling (LER)
IPL+Nd:YAG	VascuLight Elite (Lumenis)	515–200		0,5–25		3–90	35 × 8	Contact cooling/ combined with 1064
IPL+Nd:YAG	Starlux (Palomar)	400–1200	LUX-G: 500–670 and 870–1200 LUX-Y : 525–1200 LuxR: 650–1200 LuxRs: 650–1200	LuxG: 0.5–500 LuxY: 1–500 LuxR: 5–500 LuxRs: 5–500		LuxG: Up to 50 LuxY: Up to 35 LuxR: Up to 30 LuxRs:Up to 50	LuxG:12 × 12 LuxY:16?46 LuxR:16?46 LuxR:12?28	Lux 1064
IPL+Nd:YAG Xeo (Cutera)		600–850	600–850			5–20		
IPL + bipolar RF	Aurora SR (Yokneam Illit, Syneron)	580–980	580–980			Light energy 10–30 RF energy 5–20 J/cm3	12 × 25	

epidermal pigmented lesions. Furthermore, in the absence of reproducible spatial thermal injury confinement, the risk of scarring and pigmentary changes is significant in the hands of inexperienced operators.

The pigment-nonselective erbium and CO_2 lasers can be used to remove epidermal pigment effectively because of the ability to target H_2O in the epidermis. The nonspecific thermal damage leads to destruction of the lesion with denuding of the epidermis. Pigment is thus damaged as a secondary event. This destruction is followed by healing that may have some erythema and possible pigmentary and textural changes.

■ Q-Switched Lasers

The fundamental principle behind laser treatment of cutaneous pigment and tattoos is selective destruction of undesired pigment with minimal collateral damage. This destruction is achieved by the delivery of energy at the absorptive wavelength of the selected chromophore. The exposure time must also be limited so that the heat generated by the laser–tissue interaction is confined to the target.

The target chromophore of pigmented lesions is the melanosome and that of tattoos, is the insoluble, submicrometer intracellular pigments. Q-switched lasers produce pulses in the nanosecond range. These high peak power lasers deliver light with a pulse width shorter than the approximately 1-ms thermal relaxation time of the melanosomes or the tattoo ink particles. Various Q-switched lasers (532-nm frequency-doubled Q-switched Nd:YAG, 694-nm ruby, 755-nm alexandrite, 1064-nm Nd:YAG) are therefore used for the treatment of various epidermal, dermal, and mixed epidermal and dermal pigmented lesions and tattoos (Table 3.2).

To date, Q-switched lasers have been shown to treat both epidermal and dermal pigmented lesions effectively in a safe, reproducible fashion. Q-switched lasers used for the treatment of superficial pigmented lesions include the 532-nm frequency-doubled Q-switched Nd:YAG, the 694-nm ruby, and the 755-nm alexandrite lasers. Strong absorption of light at these wavelengths by melanin makes these lasers an excellent treatment modality for superficial pigmented lesions. The Q-switched 694-nm ruby, 755-nm alexandrite and 1064-nm Nd:YAG lasers are useful for treating deeper pigmented lesions such as nevus of Ota and tattoos. The Q-switched 1064 nm laser should be used when treating patients with darker skin, because it reduces the risk of epidermal injury and pigmentary alteration.

■ Pulsed-Dye Laser

The short wavelength (510 nm) and 300-ns pigment lesion dye laser (PLDL) is highly effective in the treatment of superficial, pigmented lesions and red tattoos, but is no longer commercially available.

■ Long-Pulsed Lasers

To target large, pigmented lesions, such as hair follicles or nevocellular nevi, lasers with longer (millisecond- as opposed to nanosecond-range) pulse durations are more suitable (Table 3.1). These include the long-pulsed 694-nm ruby, 755-nm alexandrite, 810-nm diode and 1064-nm Nd:YAG lasers. The millisecond pulse width more closely matches the thermal relaxation time of the hair follicles or the nested melanocytes. Collateral thermal damage results in injury to the stem cells located in the outer root sheath or the melanocytes adjacent to the target area that may actually not contain melanin. However, it is unlikely that every nevus cell is destroyed. Cautious follow-up of nevi treated with laser light is necessary.

■ Intense Pulsed Light Sources

Intense pulsed light (IPL) systems are high-intensity light sources, which emit polychromatic light (Table 3.3). Unlike lasers, these flashlamps work with noncoherent light over a broad wavelength spectrum of 515–1200 nm. Because of the wide spectrum of potential combinations of wavelengths, pulse durations, pulse intervals, and fluences, IPLs have proven to very efficiently treat photodamaged pigmented lesions like solar lentigines and generalized dyschromia.

3

Indications

There are many types of pigmented lesions. Each varies in the amount, depth, and density of melanin or tattoo ink distribution. The approach to the treatment of cutaneous pigmentation depends on the location of the pigment (epidermal, dermal, or mixed), the way it is packaged (intracellular, extracellular) and the nature of the pigment (melanin or tattoo particles). The benign pigmented lesions which do respond well to laser treatment include: lentigines, ephelides (freckles), nevus of Ota, nevus of Ito, and "blue" nevus. Varying results are obtained in café-au-lait maculae, nevus spilus, and nevus of Becker. Treatment of congenital and acquired nevi is still controversial because of the risk of incomplete destruction of deeper-situated nevus cells. Hyperpigmentation, like melasma and postinflammatory hyperpigmentation, only shows a moderate response. Finally, laser treatment in itself can result in postinflammatory hyperpigmentation.

Epidermal Pigmented Lesions

In general, epidermal pigment is easier to eradicate than dermal pigment because of its proximity to the skin's surface. Several lasers can effectively treat epidermal lesions. These include the Q-switched laser systems, pulsed visible light lasers and flashlamps, CW lasers, and

CO_2 or erbium lasers. The goal is to remove unwanted epidermal pigmentation, and as long as the injury is above the dermal-epidermal junction, it will heal without scarring.

■ Lentigo Simplex, Solar Lentigo

Lentigines are benign macular epidermal lesions caused by ultraviolet light, They contain melanin within keratinocytes and melanocytes. The superficial nature of lentigines allows the use of several lasers, including frequency-doubled Q-switched Nd:YAG, Q-switched ruby, alexandrite, Nd:YAG, pulsed 510 nm, CW argon, CO_2 or erbium, and other pulsed visible-light lasers. Labial melanocytic macules are similar lesions found on the mucosal surface and respond well to treatment with Q-switched lasers (Fig. 3.2).

Lentigines frequently clear with 1–3 treatments. The argon laser (488 nm, 514 nm), the 510-nm pigment laser, and the 532-nm green light lasers treat lentigines with superior efficacy, especially lightly pigmented lesions in which less chromophore is present. These shorter wavelength lasers are better absorbed by melanin but have less penetration. Use of a broadband sunscreen helps prevent new lentigines from occurring as well as the recurrence of treated lesions.

Correct diagnosis is a primary concern when treating lentigines. Lentigo maligna should not be treated with laser. Although initially one can obtain excellent cosmetic results,

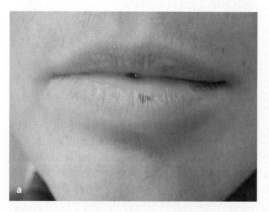
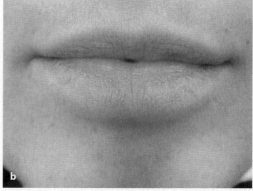

Fig. 3.2. Labial lentigo. Complete clearing after single treatment with a Q-switched alexandrite laser

recurrences are frequently seen. Lentigo maligna frequently has an amelanotic portion, which is not susceptible to laser treatment and will allow for recurrence. These cases emphasize the importance of careful clinical assessment before any laser surgery and the need to advise patients to return for evaluation if pigmentation does return.

▪ Seborrheic Keratosis

Seborrheic keratoses are benign epidermal lesions that have melanin distribution similar to lentigines and a thickened, hyperkeratotic epidermis. Liquid nitrogen cryotherapy and other surgical methods like CO_2 or erbium laser are useful in treating these lesions, but are not practical modalities to tolerate in patients who have large numbers of lesions. Using pulsed green or Q-switched lasers offer the possibility to quickly and efficiently destroy hundreds of flat pigment seborrheic keratoses.

▪ Ephelides

Ephelides or freckles are responsive to Q-switched laser treatment. Patients who tend to freckle are likely to refreckle with any sun exposure. At a follow-up of 24 months after laser treatment, 40% of patients showed partial recurrence. However, all the patients maintained >50% improvement. The use of a broad band sunscreen is therefore indicated.

▪ Café-au-Lait Macules

Café-au-lait macules are light to dark brown flat hypermelanotic lesions and may be a solitary benign finding or associated with certain genodermatoses (e. g., neurofibromatosis). Histologically, hypermelanosis is present within the epidermis and giant melanosomes may be present in both basal melanocytes and keratinocytes. Although café-au-lait macules are thin, superficial lesions, they are notoriously difficult to treat, and multiple treatments are required for even the possibility of complete eradication. There is probably a cellular influence in the dermis that triggers the pigmentation in the more superficial cells. This underlying biology may also explain why pigment recurrences are often observed. Lesions may remain clear for up to a year with spontaneous or UV-induced recurrences in more than 50% of cases. Patient education is important so that the possibility of recurrence is understood. However, given the significant disfigurement associated with many of these larger facial lesions, laser treatment is an excellent treatment option. Q-switched lasers with wavelengths of 532 nm or the pulsed 510-nm (Alster 1995) laser can adequately treat the café-au-lait macules (Fig. 3.3). Erbium laser superficial abrasion of the epidermis of a "Q-switched laser-resistant" cafe-au-lait macule has also been reported to be a successful treatment modality.

▪ Nevus Spilus

When darker-pigmented macules or papules (junctional or compound melanocytic nevi) lie within the café-au-lait macule, the lesion is called nevus spilus. The lasers used for café-au-lait macules have also been used for nevus spilus (Carpo et 1999). The darker lesions tend to respond better than the lighter café-au-lait

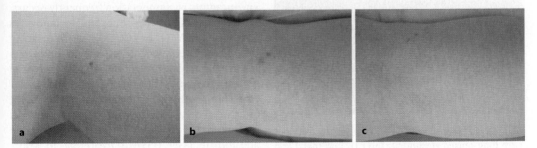

Fig. 3.3. Café-au-lait macule. Complete clearing after four treatments

macule. There can be complete removal of the junctional or compound nevus portion but no improvement in the cafe-au-lait portion. Cases of nevus spilus transformation into melanoma have been reported in the literature. These cases emphasize the need for careful clinical assessment before any laser surgery, and continued evaluation after laser treatment.

Dermal-Epidermal Pigmented Lesions

■ Becker's Nevus

Becker's nevus is an uncommon pigmented hamartoma that develops during adolescence and occurs primarily in young men. The nevus is characterized by hypertrichosis and hyperpigmentation and is usually located unilaterally over the shoulder, upper arm, scapula, or trunk. These lesions often require the use of millisecond pigment-specific lasers for treatment of the hair, but the pigment lightening is variable. Test sites with a variety a pigment-specific Q-switched and millisecond lasers or flashlamps is recommended to determine which one (or combination) will be the best treatment option (Fig. 3.4). More recently, ablation of the epidermis and superficial dermis with an erbium laser

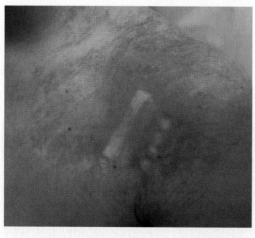

Fig. 3.4. Beckers nevus. Good clearing in test spot with long-pulsed alexandrite laser (*round spots*) and in test spot with IPL (*rectangles*)

has been shown to result in occasional complete pigment clearance with a single treatment.

■ Postinflammatory Hyperpigmentation

Treatment of postinflammatory hyperpigmentation with laser is unpredictable and often unsatisfactory. Furthermore, patients with hyperpigmentation following trauma are likely to respond to laser irradiation with an exacerbation of their pigment. The use of test sites is therefore recommended before an entire area is treated.

■ Postsclerotherapy Hyperpigmentation

Cutaneous pigmentation commonly occurs following sclerotherapy of varicose veins. Pigmentation most likely reflects hemosiderin deposition, which is secondary to extravasation of red blood cells through the damaged endothelium (Goldman et al. 1987). Hemosiderin has an absorption spectrum that peaks at 410–415 nm followed by a gradually sloping curve throughout the remainder of the visible spectrum. Several Q-switched or pulsed lasers have therefore been reported to result in significant resolution of hemosiderin pigmentation (Goldman 1987; Sanchez et al. 1981).

■ Melasma

Melasma is an acquired, usually symmetric light to dark brown facial hypermelanosis. It is associated with multiple etiologic factors (pregnancy, racial, and endocrine), and one of the primary causes of its exacerbation appears to be exposure to sunlight. Although the results after Q-switched laser treatment are usually initially encouraging, repigmentation frequently occurs.

Destruction of the abnormal melanocytes with erbium:YAG or CO_2 laser resurfacing has been attempted. It effectively improves melasma, however, there is almost universal appearance of transient postinflammatory hyperpigmentation which necessitates prompt and persistent intervention. A combination of pulsed CO_2 laser followed by Q-switched alexandrite laser (QSAL) treatment to selectively eliminate the dermal melanin with the alexandrite laser has also been examined. Combined pulsed CO_2 laser and QSAL showed a better result than CO_2 or QSAL alone, but was associated with more frequent adverse effects. Long-term follow-up and a larger number of cases are required to determine its efficacy and safety for refractory melasma.

▪ Nevocellular Nevi

Although laser treatment of many pigmented lesions is accepted, treatment of nevocellular nevi is an evolving field with much controversy. It has yet to be determined if laser treatment increases the risk of malignant transformation by irritating melanocytes or decreases it by decreasing the melanocytic load. For this reason, laser treatment of nevi should be undertaken cautiously.

▪ Congenital Melanocytic Nevi

The management of giant congenital melanocytic nevi (GCMN) remains difficult. It has been well proved that there is an increased risk of malignant changes among patients with these lesions, although the amount of increased risk for each individual patient is not clear. There is also a balance to be achieved between limiting the risk of malignant change and minimizing the disfiguring appearance of these lesions. Sometimes GCMN are too large to be removed by multiple surgical excisions or use of osmotic tissue expanders. Removal of superficial nevus cells is possible by dermabrasion, curettage, shave excision, or laser. High energy CO_2 laser therapy is less traumatic and can produce acceptable cosmetic results. Erbium laser treatment can also be used because it causes less thermal damage and faster wound healing. These techniques, although improving the cosmetic appearance, do not remove all nevus cell nests. Therefore they do not completely eliminate the risk of malignant transformation.

Treatment of giant, congenital nevi with a long-pulsed ruby laser has been reported. These systems show promise with follow-up for at least 8 years after laser treatment. There has been no evidence of malignant change in the treated areas. However, the longer laser-emitted pulse widths can lead to thermal damage of surrounding collagen with resultant scar formation. This is especially true with darker, thicker lesions with a deep dermal component, which are often the ones whose removal is most desired. Combination therapy is therefore under investigation where Q-switched or resurfacing lasers may be used first to reduce the superficial component, followed by one of the millisecond pigment-specific lasers.

▪ Congenital and Acquired Small Melanocytic Nevi

The Q-switched ruby, alexandrite, and Nd:YAG lasers have been studied for treatment of melanocytic nevi (Goldberg 1995). Although clearing rates as high as 80% have been reported, short-pulsed lasers are not recommended for nevi because of the high postlaser treatment recurrence rates. Melanocytic nevi often have nested melanocytes with significant amounts of melanin and therefore may act more as a larger body than as individual melanosomes. It has therefore been suggested that longer pulsed ruby, alexandrite, or diode lasers or Q-switched lasers in combination with longer-pulsed lasers may provide a more effective treatment with fewer recurrences. All laser systems have been partially beneficial. No lesions have had complete histologic removal of all nevomelanocytes (Duke et al. 1999).

Dermal Pigmented Lesions

The development of Q-switched lasers has revolutionized the treatment of dermal melanocytosis. The dendritic cells found deep in the dermis are particularly sensitive to short-pulsed laser light, frequently resulting in complete lesional clearing without unwanted textural changes.

▪ Nevus of Ota, Nevus of Ito

Nevus of Ota is a form of dermal melanocytic hamartoma that appears as a bluish discoloration in the trigeminal region. Histologic examination shows long, dermal melanocytes widely scattered in the upper half of the dermis. Nevus of Ito is a persistent grayish-blue discoloration with the same histologic characteristics of nevus of Ota, but is generally present on the shoulder or upper arm, in the area innervated by the posterior supraclavicular and lateral brachial cutaneous nerves.

The dermal melanocytes found within these lesions contain melanin and are highly amenable to treatment with Q-switched ruby (Geronemus 1992; Goldberg 1992), alexandrite (Alster 1995), or Nd:YAG lasers. Four to eight treatment sessions are typically required to treat these lesions. Possible side effects like postinflammatory hyperpigmentation, hypopigmentation or scarring, and recurrences are infrequent. Although there have been no reports of successful treatment of nevus of Ito, treatment with Q-switched lasers should be efficacious.

■ Blue Nevi

Blue nevi are benign melanocytic lesions that arise spontaneously in children or young adults. The melanocytes are deep within the dermis and the blue-black color results from the Tyndall light scattering effect of the overlying tissues. Although extremely rare, malignant blue nevi have been reported. Because of their benign nature, blue nevi are usually removed for cosmetic reasons. The deep dermal melanocytes respond well to Q-switched laser treatment, as long as the lesion does not extend into the deep subcutaneous tissue.

■ Acquired Bilateral Nevus of Ota-Like Macules (ABNOMs)

Acquired bilateral nevus of Ota-like macules (ABNOM), also called nevus fuscoceruleus zygomaticus or nevus of Hori, is a common Asian condition that is characterized by bluish hyperpigmentation in the bilateral malar regions. Unlike nevus of Ota, ABNOM is an acquired condition that often develops after 20 years of age, involves both sides of the face, and has no mucosal involvement. Histologically, active melanin-synthesizing dermal melanocytes are dispersed in the papillary and middle portions of the dermis. Since these lesions are histologically a form of dermal melanocytosis like nevus of Ota, melanin-targeting lasers should be effective in the treatment. Although promising results in the treatment of Hori's nevus with Q-switched ruby, alexandrite, and Nd:YAG lasers have been reported, the treatment responses have been noted to be less effective than that of nevus of Ota. Multiple laser sessions are necessary to obtain cosmetically desired improvement. A higher rate of postinflammatory hyperpigmentation is often present after laser treatments.

Tattoos

The popularity of tattoos is burgeoning with 20–30 million tattooed individuals in the Western world. Requests for removal can be expected to rise concurrently with increased applications. Despite their relatively easy acquisition, the removal of tattoos has long been a real problem. Laser removal of tattoos is potentially a more cosmetically acceptable method of removing tattoos than surgical excision or dermabrasion.

■ Tattoo Pigments

Tattoos, a form of exogenous pigment, are usually composed of multiple colors and various dyes. In contrast to drugs and cosmetics, tattoo pigments have never been controlled or regulated in any way, and the exact composition of a given tattoo pigment is often kept a "trade secret" by the manufacturer. In most cases, neither the tattoo artist nor the tattooed patient has any idea of the composition of the tattoo pigment.

Until recently, most coloring agents in tattoo pigment were inorganic heavy metal salts and oxides, like aluminum, titanium, cadmium, chromium, cobalt, copper, iron, lead, and mercury. There has been a shift in recent years away from these agents toward organic pigments, especially azo- and polycyclic compounds. These pigments are considered safer and well tolerated by the skin, although allergic reactions and phototoxicity occur.

■ Laser Removal of Tattoos

For Q-Switched laser tattoo treatment to be effective, the absorption peak of the pigment must match the wavelength of the laser energy. Similar colors may contain different pigments, with different responses to a given laser wavelength, and not all pigments absorb the wavelengths of currently available medical lasers.

Tattoos absorb maximally in the following ranges: red tattoos, from 505 to 560 nm (green spectrum); green tattoos, from 630 to 730 nm (red spectrum); and a blue-green tattoo, in two ranges from 400 to 450 nm and from 505 to 560 nm (blue-purple and green spectrums, respectively). Yellow tattoos absorbed maximally from 450 to 510 nm (blue-green spectrum), purple tattoos-absorbed maximally from 550 to 640 nm (green-yellow-orange-red spectrum), blue tattoos absorbed maximally from 620 to 730 nm (red spectrum), and orange tattoos absorbed maximally from 500 to 525 nm (green spectrum). Black and gray absorbed broadly in the visible spectrum, but these colors most effectively absorb 600- to 800-nm laser irradiation.

Three types of lasers are currently used for tattoo removal: Q-switched ruby laser (694 nm), Q-switched Nd:YAG laser (532 nm, 1064 nm), and Q-switched alexandrite (755 nm) laser (Adrian 2000). The Q-switched ruby and alexandrite lasers are useful for removing black, blue, and green pigment (Alster 1995). The Q-switched 532-nm Nd:YAG laser can be used to remove red pigments, and the 1064-nm Nd:YAG laser is used for removal of black and blue pigments (Kilmer et al. 1993). Since many wavelengths are needed to treat multicolored tattoos, not one laser system can be used alone to remove all the available inks (Kilmer 1993; Levine 1995).

There is still much to be learned about removing tattoo pigment. Once ink is implanted into the dermis, the particles are found predominantly within fibroblasts, macrophages, and occasionally as membrane-bound pigment granules.

Exposure to Q-switched lasers produces selective fragmentation of these pigment-containing cells. The pigment particles are reduced in size and found extracellularly. A brisk inflammatory response occurs within 24 h. Two weeks later, the laser-altered tattoo ink particles are found repackaged in the same type of dermal cells.

It is not yet clear how the liberated ink particles are cleared from the skin after laser treatment. Possible mechanisms for tattoo lightening include: (1) systemic elimination by phagocytosis and transport of ink particles by inflammatory cells, (2) external elimination via a scale-crust that is shed, or (3) alteration of the optical properties of the tattoo to make it less apparent. The first of these appears clinically and histologically to be the dominant mechanism.

There are five types of tattoos: professional, amateur, traumatic, cosmetic, and medicinal. In general, amateur tattoos require fewer treatment sessions than professional multicolored tattoos. Densely pigmented or decorative professional tattoos are composed of a variety of colored pigments and may be particularly difficult to remove, requiring 10 or more treatment sessions in some cases (Fig. 3.5). A 100% clearing rate is not always obtained and, in some instances, tattoos can be resistant to further treatment. Amateur tattoos are typically less dense, and are often made up of carbon-based ink that responds more readily to Q-switched laser treatment (Fig. 3.6). Traumatic tattoos usually have minimal pigment deposited superficially and often clear with a few treatments (Ashinoff 1993) (Fig. 3.7). Caution should be used when treating gunpowder or firework tattoos, because the implanted material has the potential to ignite and cause pox-like scars.

Consent

After obtaining informed consent (Fig. 3.8), the following options are considered.

Personal Laser Technique

The approach to treatment will vary with the chosen laser and whether the pigmented lesion to be treated is epidermal, dermal, or mixed. Tattoos may show a different response (Tables 3.4–3.6).

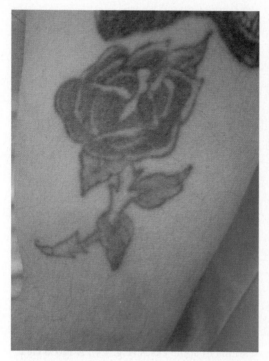
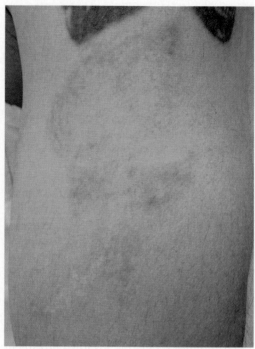

Fig. 3.5. Professional tattoo. Partial clearing after four treatments

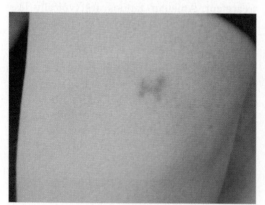
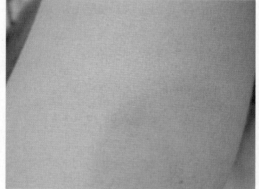

Fig. 3.6. Amateur tattoo. Complete clearing after two treatments

Q-Switched Ruby Laser (694 nm)

The first Q-switched laser developed was a ruby laser. Current models employ a mirrored articulated arm with a variable spot size of 5 or 6.5 mm, a pulse width of 28–40 ns and a maximum fluence of up to 10 J/cm². The 694-nm wavelength is most well absorbed by melanin. Because hemoglobin absorbs 694-nm light poorly, the ruby laser treats pigmented lesions very efficiently.

Most lentigines and ephelides clear after one to three treatments with the Q-switched ruby laser (QSRL). Café-au-lait macules, nevus spilus, and Becker's nevus respond moderately well. Recurrences are frequent with these

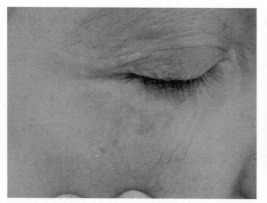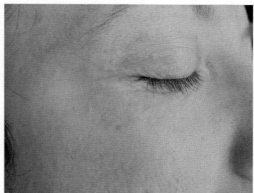

Fig. 3.7. Traumatic tattoo. Clearing after three treatments

lesions, especially when incomplete clearing is obtained. The QSRL has become the treatment of choice for dermal pigmented lesions like nevus of Ota or Ito. The long wavelength, the big spot size and the high delivered energy per pulse generates a high fluence deep in the tissue. This all leads to efficient targeting of deep melanocytes. As effective as other Q-switched lasers are for removing black tattoo ink, the QSRL is one of the better lasers for removing dark blue or green ink. Removal of red tattoo ink is problematic given that the QSRL is a red light source and is not well absorbed by the red ink particles. Yellow ink does not respond to QSRL treatment because the absorption of yellow inks is very low in this laser's red to near-infrared spectrum of delivered light.

When selecting the energy level for treatment with the QSRL, immediate tissue whitening with no or minimal tissue bleeding should be observed. The required energy level is determined by the degree of pigmentation or the amount and color of the tattoo ink. The 6.5-mm spot is recommended for most lesions, with an initial fluence of 3–5 J/cm². The excellent QSRL melanin absorption frequently leads to transient hypopigmentation, which may take months to resolve. Rarely (in 1%–5% of cases), one sees permanent depigmentation.

Q-Switched Nd:YAG Laser (532–1064 nm)

The Q-switched Nd:YAG laser (QSNd:YL) emits two wavelengths, 532 and 1064 nm, with a pulse duration of 5–10 ns, delivered through a mirrored, articulated arm. Current models have spot sizes of 2–8 mm and can operate at up to 10 Hz.

The long QSNd:YL 1064-nm wavelength has the least absorption by melanin and the deepest penetration. It is therefore potentially effective for both epidermal and dermal pigmented lesions. Use of a frequency-doubling crystal allows emission of a 532-nm wavelength (green). This wavelength is well absorbed by both melanin and hemoglobin. Because of the superficial penetration, this 532-nm laser is limited to treating epidermal pigmented lesions.

Epidermal lesions such as lentigines or ephelides treated with the QSNd:YL respond as well to treatment as they do after QSRL treatment. Café-au-lait macules, nevus spilus, and Becker's nevus do not respond as well to QSNd:YL treatment. The Q-switched 1064-nm laser is highly effective for removing deep dermal pigment such as nevus of Ota and Ito. Because this wavelength is less absorbed by melanin, higher energy is required than with the QSRL. Newly available Q-switched Nd:YAG lasers which generate high fluences at large spot sizes, have optimized treatment results. In an effort to treat tattoos without interference of melanin absorption, the 1064-nm Q- switched

CONSENT FORM FOR TREATMENT BY PIGMENT LASER

The undersigned:

Patient: . . . .

Born on: . . . . . . / . . . . . . / . . . .

Resident of . . . .

Physician: . . . .

1. INTRODUCTION
The contents of this form give a brief overview of the information exchanged and explained during the preceding oral conversations between both parties.
The patient is considered to be well informed before consenting to receiving pigment laser treatment.
   It is obvious that the treating physician is prepared to answer all your possible questions regarding this operation.

2. NATURE AND COURSE OF THE TREATMENT
The pigment laser is a device producing highly energetic light. During the treatment, a laser beam is pointed at the skin. The laser beam selectively destroys the melanin pigment or tattoo particles in the skin, while the surrounding tissues are left untouched. In general, local anesthesia is not needed. In case it should be necessary for one or another reason, the treating physician will discuss the modalities thereof in detail. During laser treatment, the patient, the physician and the personnel are to wear special glasses to protect the eyes against the laser light.

3. AIM OF THE TREATMENT
The aim of the treatment is to clear up a lesion caused by melanin pigment or tattoo particles. The number of treatments depends on the extent, the nature, the age and the intensity of the pigmentation of the skin lesion. A complete disappearance of the treated lesion is aimed at, but can never be guaranteed in advance.
   The physician thus agrees with the patient to operate according to the rules of art, but cannot promise any well-defined result (= commitment to make every possible effort).

4. RISKS
Potential complications of the treatment are:
– Wound infection: occurs very rarely and heals when treated appropriately.
– Formation of scar tissue: highly exceptional.
– Increased or decreased pigmentation:
In some cases, the wound heals with increased pigmentation (hyperpigmentation). This usually happens among patients with darker skin tones or as a result of sun exposure. Other patients are predestined to have this kind of reaction and may have experienced this before, during the healing of other wounds. In order to minimize the risk of hyperpigmentation, post-operational protection of the skin against sun exposure is of the utmost importance. Among some patients, this hyperpigmentation can even occur despite good sun protection. Hyperpigmentation is usually only temporary, but needs a few months to clear. Seldom does the hyperpigmentation persist nevertheless.
Among some patients, the treated area may show decreased pigmentation (hypopigmentation) and thus obtain a lighter color than the surrounding skin tissue. This is usually only a temporary reaction, after which the skin will gradually pigment again. In some cases, however, the depigmentation may be permanent.
The physician has informed the patient how to take care of the treated skin area. Not following these postoperative instructions may cause complications.

Fig. 3.8. Consent form

5. EFFECTS

Immediately after being treated, the skin will turn whitish gray. Exceptionally, erosion (superficial wound) and/or pinpoint bleeding may occur. A bluish red discoloration as a consequence of bleeding may also appear and may last up to 2 weeks before disappearing.

6. ALTERNATIVE TREATMENTS

Cryotherapy, excisional surgery and dermabrasion are possible alternatives.

7. PHOTOGRAPHS

In order to have a better view on the results of the operation, and for educational and scientific purposes, such as presentations and scientific publications, photographs may possibly be taken. The patient will be turned unrecognizable on these pictures. The patient is well informed about this and agrees to it.

8. REVOCATION OF CONSENT

The patient deliberately consents to the treatment and can at any moment decide to stop further treatment.

9. OBSERVATIONS

Observations of the physician:

. . . .
. . . .
. . . .

Observations of the patient:

. . . .
. . . .
. . . .
. . . .

10. Each of the consenting parties declares to have received a copy of this consent form. The signature is preceded by the self-written formula 'read and approved'.
The patient declares that all his/her questions have been answered.

Date: . . . .

. . . .
Patient's signature   Physician's signature

Fig. 3.8. Consent form (continued)

Nd:YAG laser was developed. It is most effective for treating black ink tattoos, especially in darker skin types. The 532-nm wavelength is the treatment of choice for red tattoo pigment.

When treating epidermal pigmented lesions with the 532-nm wavelength, nonspecific vascular injury will occur, leading to purpura, which takes 5–10 days to resolve. Because of the ultrashort pulse duration, the Q-switched Nd:YAG laser produces the greatest amount of epidermal debris. This can be minimized by the use of larger spot sizes. Recent studies have shown that larger spot sizes and lower fluences are as effective in removing tattoo pigment as smaller spot sizes at higher fluences, and have fewer side effects. Therefore, when using the 1064-nm wavelength, treatment should begin with a 4- to 8-mm spot size at 3–6 J/cm^2.

3

Table 3.4. Suggested treatment parameters for pigmented lesions

Indication	Laser	Spot size(mm)	Fluence (J/cm²)
Lentigines	510-nm PLPD	3	2.5
	QS 532-nm Nd:YAG	4	3
	QS 694-nm ruby	6.5	3–5
	QS 755-nm alexandrite	4	3.4
Café-au-lait macules	510-nm PLPD	5	2–3.5
	QS 532-nm Nd:YAG	3	1–1.5
	QS 694-nm ruby	6.5	3–4.5
	QS 755-nm alexandrite	3	4–5
Becker's nevus	QS 532-nm Nd:YAG	3	1.5–2
	QS 694-nm ruby	6.5	4.5
	QS 755-nm alexandrite	3	6
	QS 1064-nm Nd:YAG	3	4–5
Nevus Spilus	QS 532-nm Nd:YAG	3	1.5–2
	QS 694-nm ruby	6.5	4.5
	QS 755-nm alexandrite	3	6
	QS 1064-nm Nd:YAG	3	4–5
Tattoo	510-nm PLPD	5	2–3.5
	QS 532-nm Nd:YAG	3	2–3.5
	QS 694-nm ruby	6.5	5–8
	QS 755-nm alexandrite	3	6–6.5
	QS 1064-nm Nd:YAG	3	5–8
Nevus of Ota	QS 694-nm ruby	6.5	5–6
	QS 755-nm alexandrite	3	6.5
	QS 1064-nm Nd:YAG	3	5.0

Table 3.5. Most effective Q-switched lasers for different tattoo ink colors

Tattoo ink color	Laser
Blue/black	Q-switched ruby, Q-switched alexandrite, Q-switched 1064-nm Nd:YAG
Green	Q-switched ruby, Q-switched alexandrite
Red/orange/purple	Q-switched frequency-doubled 532-nm Nd:YAG laser, 510-nm pigment lesion pulsed dye laser

Table 3.6. Response of pigmented lesions and tattoos to various lasers and light sources

| | Pigmented Lesions | | Tattoos | | |
	Epidermal	Mixed	Dermal	Amateur	Professional
510-nm pigment lesion pulsed dye laser	+++	+	+	++	+++ (red colors)
532-nm Q-switched Nd:YAG laser	+++	+	+	++	+++ (red colors)
694-nm Q-switched ruby laser	+++	+	+++	+++	+++ (green colors)
755-nm Q-switched alexandrite laser	+++	+	++	+++	+++ (green colors)
1064-nm Q-switched Nd:YAG laser	++	+	+++	+++	+++
Intense pulsed Light source	+++	+	+		

+++ = excellent, ++ = good, + = fair

Q-Switched Alexandrite Laser (755 nm)

The alexandrite laser has a wavelength of 755 nm, a pulse duration of 50–100 ns, a spot size of 2–4 mm and is delivered by a fiberoptic arm. Fiberoptic delivery allows a more even beam profile with fewer hot spots.

The wavelength of the Q-switched alexandrite laser (QSAL) is similar enough to that of the QSRL to obtain comparable results for the treatment of epidermal and dermal pigmented lesions, perhaps with the added advantage of a slightly deeper penetration. Similar to the QSRL, this laser is effective at removing black, blue, and most green tattoo inks, and less proficient at removing red or orange inks.

Depending on the spot size, a starting fluence of 5–6 J/cm² is usually employed. Immediately after treatment, gray-whitening of the skin occurs, followed by erythema and edema. There is a lower risk of tissue splatter because of the longer pulse duration and the more even beam profile. There is also a lower risk of transient hypopigmentation because of slightly less QSAL melanin absorption as compared to the QSRL.

Pulsed Dye Laser (510 nm)

The short wavelength of the pulsed dye laser (PDL) makes it optimal for treatment of superficial pigmented lesions. Epidermal lesions such as lentigines, ephelides, and flat, pigmented seborrheic keratoses respond extremely well to the 510-nm pulsed dye laser. Its shallow depth of penetration into the skin makes it less than ideal for treating dermal pigmented lesions. However, like the frequency-doubled 532-nm Nd:YAG laser, the 510-nm PDL laser effectively removes bright tattoo colors like red, purple, and orange.

Continuous Wave (CW) Lasers

The CW argon (488 and 514 nm), CW dye (577 and 585 nm), CW krypton (521–530 nm), and the pulse train quasi-CW copper vapor lasers (510 and 578 nm) all have been used to treat pigmented lesions. However, when these lasers are used in freehand mode, reproducibility is lacking and the thermal damage is somewhat unpredictable. The risk of scarring and pigmentary changes is therefore significant in the hands of inexperienced operators. In general, these CW lasers, when used by skilled operators, are effective in the treatment of epidermal pigmented lesions.

CO₂ and Erbium Lasers

The CO_2 and erbium lasers are sources that emit infrared (IR) light at a wavelength of 10,600 nm and 2940 nm, respectively. These wavelengths are well absorbed by water. The lasers destroy the superficial skin layers nonselectively and can be used to remove superficial epidermal pigment, especially seborrheic keratoses. Superficial erbium laser epidermal abrasion of a "Q-switched laser-resistant" cafe-au-lait macule has also been reported. Theses ablative lasers can also be helpful in treating resistant tattoos by removing the epidermis immediately before Q-switched laser treatment. This will lead to facilitated transepidermal tattoo particle elimination.

Intense Pulsed Light (IPL) Sources

Melanin pigmentation, as part of photo aging, can be epidermal or dermal. It is often a combination of both. In early solar damage, melasma is a regular constituent; often with both dermal and epidermal pigment deposition. In later stages of solar degeneration the solar lentigo, which is mainly located in the epidermis, is a prominent feature. Recently, intense pulsed light sources (IPL) have shown to be highly effective in the treatment of photodamaged pigmented lesions like solar lentigines, and generalized dyschromia (Fig. 3.9). Unfortunately, light spectra, pulse duration, and number of pulses as well as delivered fluence and the use of skin cooling vary considerably among the published investigations, making direct comparisons of IPL devices quite difficult.

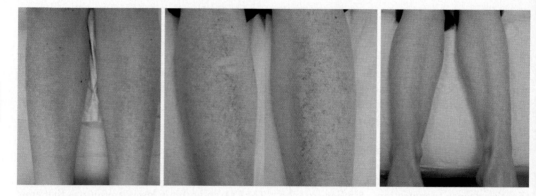

Fig. 3.9. Actinic bronzing. Sloughing of pigment 2 days after treatment. Complete clearance 1 month after treatment

Further Treatment Pearls

When treating pigmented lesions and tattoos, the laser handpiece should be held perpendicular over the area to be treated. Pulses should be delivered with 0–10% overlap until the entire lesion is treated.

The desired laser tissue interaction produces immediate whitening of the treated area with minimal or no epidermal damage or pinpoint bleeding. It is best to use the largest spot size to minimize epidermal damage. If epidermal debris is significant, the fluence should be lowered. Higher fluences may be needed with subsequent treatments when less pigment or tattoo ink particles are still present in the skin.

IPL treatment or Q-switched laser treatment of epidermal pigmented lesions rarely requires anesthesia. When needed, a topical anesthetic cream can be applied 1–2 hours before the procedure to reduce the discomfort. For more complete anesthesia, local anesthetic infiltration or regional nerve block can be used.

Treatment parameters are determined by the type of lesion and the patient's skin type. As discussed above, the ideal response is immediate whitening of the skin with little or no epidermal disruption. If the fluence is too low, the whitening will be minimal, whereas if the fluence is too high, the epidermis is ruptured and bleeding might occur. Following treatment with a 510-nm PDL or a QS 532-nm laser, pinpoint bleeding usually appears and lasts for 7–10 days. This occurs because of vessel rupture after hemoglobin absorption.

The whitening of the treated area lasts about 15 minutes and an urticarial reaction appears around the treated area. In the following days, the treated area usually becomes darker and develops a crust that falls off in 7–10 days (Fig. 3.10). The postoperative care consists of application of a healing ointment, and avoidance of sun exposure, in an effort to reduce the risk of postinflammatory hyperpigmentation.

Patients with darker skin types should be treated at lower fluences. Their threshold response will occur at lower fluences than is seen with patients with lighter skin types. Treatment of suntanned individuals should be avoided because of the high risk of laser-induced hypopigmentation.

While one to three treatments are sufficient to treat most lentigines, multiple treatments will be necessary for pigmented birthmarks like café-au-lait macules.

Anesthesia is rarely required for dermal pigmented lesions. When treating larger areas, topical or intralesional anesthesia may be necessary. When treating nevus of Ota, regional nerve blocks usually provide adequate anesthesia.

Treatment parameters are again determined by the type of lesion and the patient's skin type. In general, higher fluences are necessary than those required for the treatment of epidermal lesions. The threshold response should be

Fig. 3.10.
Crusting 1 week after laser
treatment of tattoo

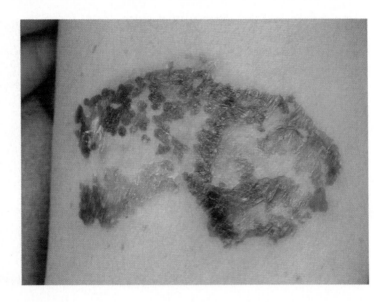

immediate whitening of the skin with little or no epidermal disruption. The same postoperative aftercare and precautions apply as for epidermal pigmented lesions. Dermal melanocytosis require multiple treatment sessions, usually performed at 6-week intervals or longer. Lesions as nevus of Ota continue to lighten for several months after each treatment.

Anesthesia is usually not required for small tattoos. For certain individuals or for larger tattoos, topical or intralesional anesthesia might be necessary.

If adequate fluences are available, it is best to use the largest laser spot size. This will reduce backward scattering and therefore minimize epidermal rupture. Following treatment, wound care is required to help healing and prevent infection. An antibiotic ointment should be applied. A dressing should be worn for several days until healing has been completed.

Tattoo treatment usually requires multiple treatments to obtain adequate clearing. Amateur tattoos respond more quickly than do multicolored professional tattoos. Complete clearing of tattoos is not always possible. During the initial consultation, the patient should be informed about this. However, dramatic lightening can be expected.

Cosmetic tattoos should be approached with caution. When treating tattoos with colors that may darken (white, light pink, tan, or some brown colors), a single test spot should be performed to assess immediate darkening (Fig. 3.11, 3.12). If darkening occurs, the same test site should be retreated to be sure the ink can be lightened before proceeding further. Although

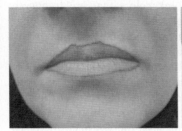 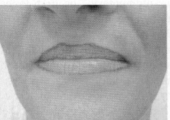 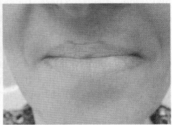

Fig. 3.11. Cosmetic tattoo. Darkening of pigment after first treatment. Partial clearing after 6 treatments with Q-switched alexandrite laser

Fig. 3.12.
Color shift to green after laser test with Q-switched alexandrite laser

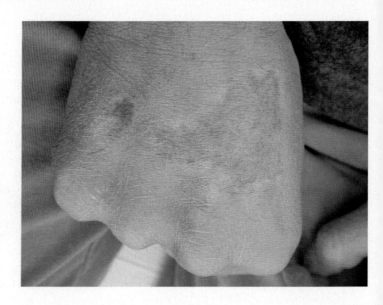

the darkened pigment may clear easily, it can sometimes be very recalcitrant to treatment. In this case, CO_2 or erbium:YAG laser vaporization can be used, as an adjunctive treatment modality, by removing the epidermis immediately before Q-switched laser treatment and/or by facilitating transepidermal tattoo particle elimination.

Treatment sessions are performed at intervals of 6 weeks or greater. Waiting longer between treatment sessions might be even more beneficial as tattoos may continue to clear for several months following each treatment.

Complications

Unlike previous treatment modalities for pigmented lesions, Q-switched lasers induce minimal side effects. These include pigmentary changes, partial removal, infection, bleeding, textural changes, and tattoo ink darkening.

Pigmentary changes following laser treatment of pigmented lesions are not uncommon. Transient hypopigmentation is most common after treatment with the 694- or 755-nm wavelengths because absorption by melanin is so strong. Permanent hypopigmentation can be seen with repetitive treatment sessions, particularly at higher fluences. The 1064-nm wavelength is the least injurious to melanocytes and is therefore the treatment of choice for dark-skinned individuals undergoing laser tattoo treatment. Transient hyperpigmentation, which has been reported in up to 15% of cases, is more common in darker skin types or following sun exposure (Kilmer et al. 1993). The incidence of scarring is less than 5%. It is associated with the use of excessive fluences. It is also more common when certain areas like the chest and ankle are treated. This complication has also been observed in areas with dense deposition of ink, such as in double tattoos. Larger laser spot sizes tend to minimize epidermal damage and are associated with fewer textural changes.

Pigment darkening of cosmetic skin color tattoos can occur after exposure to any Q-switched laser. The darkening occurs immediately and is most often seen with the red, white, or flesh-toned ink colors that are frequently used in cosmetic tattoos. These colors often contain ferric oxide and titanium dioxide that can change to a blue-black color after Q-switched laser treatment. The mechanism probably involves, at least for some tattoos, reduction of ferric oxide (Fe_2O_3, "rust") to ferrous oxide (FeO, jet black). Recently, multiple color changes following laser therapy of cosmetic tattoos has been reported (Fig. 3.11). Performing small test areas before complete treatment and using several laser wavelengths throughout the course of therapy are essential to the successful treatment of cosmetic tattoos.

Localized allergic reactions can occur with almost any treated tattoo color. It can result in an immediate hypersensitivity reaction such as urticaria (Ashinoff 1993). In the alternative, a delayed hypersensitivity reaction such as granuloma formation may occur. The most serious complication reported after Q-switched laser tattoo removal was a systemic allergic reaction. The Q-switched laser targets intracellular tattoo pigment, causing rapid thermal expansion that fragments pigment-containing cells and causes the pigment to become extracellular. This extracellular pigment may then be recognized by the immune system as foreign, potentially triggering an allergic reaction. Therefore, if a patient exhibits a local immediate hypersensitivity reaction, prophylaxis before subsequent laser treatments with systemic antihistamines and steroids should be considered. Pulsed CO_2 and erbium lasers do not seem to trigger this reaction, since the particle size does not change. These lasers may be used to enhance transepidermal elimination of ink.

Future Developments

Noninvasive, real-time optical diagnostic tools (like optical coherence tomography, confocal microscopy, multispectral digital imaging, polarized multispectral imaging) are being studied for their role in the accurate prelaser diagnosis of pigmented lesions as well as a tool for determining efficacy and safety following treatment.

Current tattoo laser research is focused on newer picosecond lasers. The systems may be more successful than the Q-switched lasers in the removal of tattoo inks (Ross 1998). Such lasers, because they emit picosecond pulse widths, cause optimal photomechanical disruption of the tattoo ink particles. Another tattoo approach would be the development of laser-responsive inks. In this case, tattoo removal might be feasible with only one or two treatment sessions.

It is also possible that a laser that emits trains of low-fluence, submicrosecond pulses might cause even more selective injury to pigmented cells by limiting mechanical damage modes. The use of pulse trains, specifically designed to selectively affect pigmented cells in skin, has not yet been tested.

Since the clearing of tattoo pigment following laser surgery is influenced by the presence of macrophages at the site of treatment, it has also been suggested that the adjuvant use of cytokines like macrophage colony-stimulating factor, other chemotactic factors such as topical leukotrienes, or the use of a topical immunomodulators like imiquimod might recruit additional macrophages to the treatment site. This could expedite the removal of tattoo pigment following laser surgery.

The extraction of magnetite ink tattoos by a magnetic field has been investigated after Q-switched laser treatment. When epidermal injury was present, a magnetic field, applied immediately after Q-switched ruby laser treatment, did extract some ink. Magnetically-extractable tattoos may therefore become feasible one day. Delivery of intradermally-focused, small energy nanosecond laser pulses might become another approach for more efficient and safer tattoo removal. Finally, optical clearing of skin with hyperosmotic chemical agents is currently under investigation. This approach reduces optical scattering in the skin, thereby enhancing the effective light dose that reaches the tattoo particles.

References

Adrian RM, Griffin L (2000) Laser tattoo removal. Clin Plast Surg 27(2):181–192

Alster TS (1995) Q-switched alexandrite laser treatment (755 nm) of professional and amateur tattoos. J Am Acad Dermatol 33(1):69–73

Anderson R, Parrish J (1983) Selective photothermolysis: precise microsurgery by selective absorption of pulsed radiation. Science 220:524–526

Ashinoff R, Levine VJ, Soter NA (1995) Allergic reactions to tattoo pigment after laser treatment. Dermatol Surg 21(4):291–294

Carpo BG, Grevelink JM, Grevelink SV (1999) Laser treatment of pigmented lesions in children. Semin Cutan Med Surg 18(3):233–243

Duke D, Byers HR, Sober AJ, Anderson RR, Grevelink JM (1999) Treatment of benign and atypical nevi with the normal-mode ruby laser and the Q-switched ruby laser: clinical improvement but failure to completely eliminate nevomelanocytes. Arch Dermatol 135(3):290–296

Geronemus RG (1992) Q-switched ruby laser therapy of nevus of Ota. Arch Dermatol 128(12):1618–1622

Goldberg DJ, Nychay S (1992) Q-switched ruby laser treatment of nevus of Ota. J Dermatol Surg Oncol 18(9):817–821

Goldberg DJ, Stampien T (1995) Q-switched ruby laser treatment of congenital nevi. Arch Dermatol 131(5):621–623

Goldman MP, Kaplan RP, Duffy DM (1987) Postsclerotherapy hyperpigmentation: a histologic evaluation. J Dermatol Surg Oncol 13(5):547–550

Kilmer SL (2002) Laser eradication of pigmented lesions and tattoos. Dermatol Clin 20(1):37–53

Kilmer Sl, Casparian JM, Wimberly JM et al (1993) Hazards of Q-switched lasers. Lasers Surg Med S5:56

Levine VJ, Geronemus RG (1995) Tattoo removal with the Q-switched ruby laser and the Q-switched Nd:YAGlaser: a comparative study. Cutis 55(5): 291–296

Ross V, Naseef G, Lin G, Kelly M, Michaud N, Flotte TJ, Raythen J, Anderson RR (1998) Comparison of responses of tattoos to picosecond and nanoseconds Q-switched neodymium: YAG lasers. Arch Dermatol 134(2):167–171

Sanchez NP, Pathak MA, Sato S, Fitzpatrick TB, Sanchez JL, Mihm MC Jr (1981) Melasma: a clinical, light microscopic, ultrastructural, and immunofluorescence study. J Am Acad Dermatol 4(6):698–710

Laser Treatment of Unwanted Hair

David J. Goldberg, Mussarrat Hussain

4

> ## Core Messages
>
> - A wide variety of lasers can now induce permanent changes in unwanted hair.
> - Hair removal lasers are distinguished not only by their emitted wavelengths, but also by their delivered pulse durations, peak fluences, spot size delivery systems, and associated cooling.
> - Nd:YAG lasers with effective cooling represent the safest approach for the treatment of darker skin.
> - Complications from laser hair removal are more common in darker skin types.
> - Pain during laser hair removal is generally a heat-related phenomenon and is multifactorial.
> - Laser treatment of nonpigmented hairs remains a challenge.

History

Human hair, its amount and distribution, plays an important role in defining appearance in contemporary society. Hair also functions in many mammals as a sensory organ, reduces friction in certain anatomic sites, protects against the environment by providing thermal insulation and thermoregulation, aids in pheromone dissemination, and plays both social and sexual roles (Wheeland 1997).

Individuals, seeking consultation for the removal of unwanted body hair, generally have increased hair in undesirable locations secondary to genetics or medical conditions. These individuals may be classified as having hirsutism or hypertrichosis. More commonly, those seeking hair removal have hair that would be considered normal in distribution and density. However, these individuals, for emotional, social, cultural, cosmetic, or other reasons, want the hair to be removed.

There has always been the need for an ideal method of hair removal that is both practical and effective. Traditional hair removal techniques have included shaving, waxing, tweezing, chemical depilation, and electrolysis.

In the early twentieth century, radiograph machines were widely used for removal of facial hair in women. Unfortunately, these treatments were associated with a high risk of complications and the potential for subsequent treatment-induced carcinogenesis.

Maiman, using a ruby crystal in 1960, developed stimulated laser emission of a 694-nm red light. This was the first working laser, and it is from this prototype that today's lasers are derived. Since 1960, research and technical advances have led to modern day lasers. Leon Goldman, the father of laser surgery, published preliminary results on the effects of a ruby laser for the treatment of skin diseases. Ohshiro et al. noted hair loss from nevi after treatment with a ruby laser (Ohshiro et al. 1983).

Early reports described the use of a CO_2 laser to eliminate unwanted hair on flaps used for pharyngoesophageal procedures. A continuous-wave Nd:YAG laser has also been shown to remove hair in urethral grafts All of this early work described lasers using ablative techniques with the effect of nonspecific vaporization of skin cells. These methods are not commonly used for hair removal today because of their limited effectiveness as well as their commonly induced permanent pigmentary changes and scarring.

Selective Photothermolysis

A detailed understanding of laser-tissue interaction emerged in 1983 as the theory of selective photothermolysis was conceived for the laser treatment of pediatric port wine stains (Anderson et al. 1983)

The theory of selective photothermolysis led to the concept of a laser-induced injury confined to microscopic sites of selective light absorption in the skin, such as blood vessels, pigmented cells, and unwanted hair with minimal damage to the adjacent tissues. To achieve this selective effect, lasers would need to fulfill three requirements:

1. They should emit a wavelength that is highly absorbed by the targeted structure.
2. They should produce sufficiently high energies to inflict thermal damage to the target.
3. The time of tissue exposure to the laser should be short enough to limit the damage to the target without heat diffusion to the surrounding tissues. This is known as the thermal relaxation time (TRT).

These concepts revolutionized cutaneous laser treatment and led to the development of successful laser and light-based hair removal devices.

Extended Theory of Selective Photothermolysis

The concept of selective photothermolysis (Anderson et al. 1983) emphasizes both the selective damage and minimum light energy requirements seen with current laser technology. However, the use of such a short pulse width laser system may become inapplicable when the target absorption is nonuniform over a treatment area. This may be seen when the actual target exhibits weak or no absorption, yet other surrounding portions of the target exhibit significant absorption. If this is the case, the weakly absorbing part of the target chromophore has

to be damaged by heat diffusion from the highly pigmented/strongly absorbing portion of the chromophore (the heater or absorber). Such nonspecific thermal damage evokes the concept of thermal damage time (TDT). The TDT of a target is the time required for irreversible target damage with sparing of the surrounding tissue. For a nonuniformly absorbing target structure, the TDT is the time it takes for the outermost part of the target to reach a target damage temperature through heat diffusion from the heated chromophore.

According to the concept of extended selective photothermolysis, target damage can still be selective even though the TDT is many times as long as the thermal relaxation time (TRT) of the actual target.

This new extended theory of selective thermal damage of nonuniformly pigmented structures in biological tissue postulates that the target is destroyed by heat diffusion from the absorbing chromophore to the target but not by direct heating from laser irradiation, as is seen with selective photothermolysis. This theory has now been applied to the treatment of unwanted hair. Ultimately, the use of hair removal lasers expanded rapidly with the subsequent development of appropriate cooling devices that minimized epidermal injury.

Physical Basis of Laser Hair Removal

Successful treatment of unwanted hair is dependent on an understanding of the optical properties of the skin. It is these properties that determine the behavior of light within the hair shaft and bulb, including the relative amount of absorption of incoming photons.

Different physical factors including delivered fluence, wavelength, pulse duration, and spot size diameter play an important role in maximizing the efficacy and safety of laser-assisted hair removal.

For optimal laser hair removal, one needs to use an optimal set of laser parameters based on anatomic and physical principles. This is determined by a time–temperature combination with the ultimate effect being transfollicular denaturation.

Pulse Duration

Laser pulse width seems to play an important role in laser-assisted hair removal. Thermal conduction during the laser pulse heats a region around each microscopic site of optical energy absorption. The spatial scale of thermal confinement and resultant thermal or thermomechanical damage is therefore strongly related to the laser pulse width. Q-switched laser nanosecond pulses effectively damage individual pigment cells within a hair follicle by confinement of heat at the spatial level of melanosomes (Zenzie et al. 2000). They can induce leukotrichia and cause a temporary hair growth delay, but do not inactivate the follicle itself.

On the other hand, lasers with longer pulse durations not only allow gentle heating of the melanosomes, but also target the entire follicular epithelium by allowing thermal conduction from the pigmented hair shaft and pigmented epithelial cells to the entire follicular structure.

Therefore, lasers emitting longer pulse durations can achieve two goals: (1) Epidermal melanosomes are preserved. This then helps to preserve the epidermis. (2) Adequate heat diffusion occurs to the surrounding follicle from the light-absorbing melanized bulb and shaft.

The use of a longer laser-emitted pulse width may necessitate the use of higher fluences because the longer pulse now heats a larger volume of tissue. This may be of some benefit in allowing higher fluences to be used on dark skin types with both less risk of epidermal injury and increased chances of transfollicular damage.

Spot Size

Large diameter laser exposure spots (e.g., >10 mm) are associated with substantially less loss of energy intensity with depth of dermal penetration as compared to small-diameter exposure spots. This is because optical scattering by dermal collagen causes light to diffuse as it penetrates into the dermis. The larger the spot, the less is the associated scattering.

Fluence

In general, higher-delivered laser fluences lead to better laser hair removal results. However, the higher the utilized fluence, the greater the discomfort and risk of complications. The effective fluence for any one area of hair is determined mainly by hair color, whereas the tolerated fluence is determined mainly by skin color.

The tolerance fluence can be increased substantially by various means, such as cooling the skin surface before, during, and/or after the optical pulse.

Factors Affecting Efficacy/Results

Hair Color

Hair color is genetically determined, and is a result of both the type and amount of melanin within the hair shaft. Melanin production occurs only during the anagen phase, by melanocytes in the bulb that transfer melanin granules to hair keratinocytes. Distinct types of melanosomes exist in hair of different colors. Dark hair contains large numbers of eumelanin granules, whereas light hair contains mostly pheomelanin. Red hair contains erythromelanin granules that are rich in pheomelanin. In gray hair, melanocytes show degenerative changes such as vacuoles and poorly melanized melanosomes, whereas in white hair melanocytes are greatly reduced in number or are absent.

Most individuals demonstrate greater melanin density in their hair as compared to their skin epidermis such that the absorption coefficient of the hair shaft and bulb is roughly 2–6 times that of the epidermis. Thus, hair will generally absorb more of the melanin-absorbing wavelengths emitted from today's laser and light source hair removal systems.

Thus, color contrast between the epidermis and the hair shaft are paramount in determining the optimal wavelengths and pulse duration for successful treatment. For high contrast (dark hair and light skin) high fluences, shorter wavelengths, and relatively short pulse durations can be used without risking epidermal injury. Conversely, low contrast areas (dark hair and dark skin) require lower fluences, longer wavelengths, and longer pulse durations for safe treatment.

Growth Centers of Hairs

The hair follicle is a self-regenerating structure and contains a population of stem cells capable of reproducing themselves. It has been noted, at least in animal models, that a complete hair follicle can be regenerated even after the matrix-containing hair follicle is surgically removed. Although the dermal papilla is not technically part of the actual hair, it remains a very important site for future hair induction, and melanin production in terminal hairs.

Long-term hair removal has been traditionally thought to require that a laser or light source impact on one or more growth centers of hair. The major growth centers have always been thought to be in the hair matrix. However, research evaluating growth of new hair has revealed that the matrix is not the only growth center. New hairs may evolve from the dermal papilla, follicular matrix, or the "bulge." These stem cells are usually found in a well-protected, highly vascularized and innervated area, often in close proximity to a population of rapidly proliferating cells. They always remain intact and, in fact, are left behind after hair plucking. Stem cells are relatively undifferentiated both ultrastructurally and biochemically. They have a large proliferative potential, and are responsible for the long-term maintenance and regeneration of the hair-generating tissue. They can be stimulated to proliferate in response to wounding and certain growth stimuli.

Hair Cycle

All human hairs show various stages of hair growth. The hair cycle is divided into three stages: anagen, the period of activity or growth phase; catagen, the period of regression or regression phase; and telogen, the period of quiescence or resting phase.

Anagen growth phase varies greatly (and can last up to 6 years) depending on age, season, anatomic region, sex, hormonal levels, and certain genetic predispositions. It is these variations that have led to the tremendous disparity in hair cycles reported by various investigators.

The catagen stage is relatively constant and is generally of 3 weeks duration, whereas the telogen phase usually lasts approximately 3 months.

The overall length of the hair is determined primarily by the duration of the anagen phase. Human hair appears to grow continuously, because the growth cycles of different hair follicles are in dysynchrony with each other.

The histologic appearance of a hair follicle also differs dramatically with the stages of growth. The anagen follicle penetrates deepest in the skin, typically to the level of subcutaneous fat. Catagen is characterized by pyknotic changes in the nuclei of the kerotinocytes, followed by apoptosis of the transient portion of the follicle. The entire transient portion (which begins at the level of the insertion of arrector pili muscle and extends to the deepest portion) is absorbed, except for the basement membrane. As the new anagen progresses, the secondary hair germ descends, enlarges, and begin to produce a hair shaft.

Although reports of anagen duration, telogen duration, and the percentage of telogen hairs represent an inexact science, most discussions of laser hair removal take into account different anatomic areas in terms of anagen and telogen cycles.

It is the sensitivity of the anagen hair to a variety of destructive processes, including laser and light source damage, that leads to a metabolic disturbance of the mitotically active anagen matrix cells. The response pattern is dependent both on the duration and intensity of the insult.

Lin et al. (Lin et al. 1998) postulate that follicles treated in the telogen phase show only a growth delay for weeks, whereas, when those follicles are treated in the anagen phase they may be susceptible to lethal damage, may have a growth delay, or may simply switch into telogen phase. This could partly explain the growth dynamics of the hair cycle. Repeated treatments could lead to a synchronization of the anagen phase by induction and/or shortening of the telogen phase, which could increase the effectiveness of hair removal with each consecutive treatment. Another explanation might be that the follicle is not destroyed immediately, but shows a growth arrest after only one (shortened) anagen cycle. Some have questioned the assumption that effective laser hair removal is determined solely by treating hairs in the anagen cycle. These investigators suggest that melanin within a hair follicle may be more important than the actual time of treatment.

Cooling

Laser hair removal-associated epidermal cooling can be achieved by various means, including ice, a cooled gel layer, a cooled glass chamber, a cooled sapphire or copper window, a pulsed cryogen spray, or solid air flow.

Epidermal melanin and melanized hairs present competing sites for absorption of light energy. Selective cooling is essential to effectively minimize photothermal-induced epidermal adverse effects. In addition, epidermal cooling also permits higher fluences to be delivered to the treated follicular structures. Ideally, the epidermal temperature should be significantly but harmlessly decreased by the cooling procedure, while the target follicular temperature should remain unchanged or changed insignificantly. If this condition is not met, the laser fluences must be increased to compensate for the lower target temperature.

Age

In an isolated study a significant negative correlation was noted between successful hair removal and the age of the patients, suggesting that hair removal was more effective in younger patients. However, other studies on hair removal have not found age to be a factor in determining efficacy.

Hormones

A number of hormones affect hair growth, with thyroid and growth hormones producing a generalized increased growth in hair. Estrogens have only minimal effects on hair growth. Androgens are the most important determinant of the type of hair distributed throughout the body. The principal circulating androgen, testosterone, is converted in the hair follicle by 5-alpha reductase to dihydrotestosterone (DHT), which stimulate the dermal papilla to produce a terminal melanized hair. The effect of androgens on hair growth is skin area-specific, due to local variations in androgen receptor and 5-alpha reductase content). While the effect of androgens on hairs (i. e., terminalization of vellus hairs) will be more readily apparent in skin areas with a greater numbers of hair follicles, hair follicle density does not correlate with follicular sensitivity to androgens. Some areas of the body, termed nonsexual skin (e. g., that of the eyelashes, eyebrows, and lateral and occipital aspects of the scalp), are relatively independent of the effect of androgens.

Other areas are quite sensitive to androgens. In these locations hair follicles are terminalized even in the presence of relatively low levels of androgens. Such areas include the pubic area and the axilla, which begin to develop terminal hair even in early puberty when only minimally increased amounts of androgens are observed. Finally, some areas of skin respond only to high levels of androgens. These sites include the chest, abdomen, back, thighs, upper arms, and face. The presence of terminal hairs in these areas is characteristically masculine, and if present in women is considered pathological, i.e., hirsutism.

Hirsutism is defined as the presence in women of terminal hairs in a male-like pattern. This affects between 5% and 10% of surveyed women. Hirsutism above all else should be principally considered a sign of an underlying endocrine or metabolic disorder, and these patients should undergo a thorough evaluation. The hormonal therapy of hirsutism consists of medications that either suppress androgen production, or block androgen action.

The main purpose of hormonal therapy is to stop new hairs from growing and potentially slow the growth of terminal hairs already present. Although hormonal therapy alone will sometimes produce a thinning and loss of pigmentation of terminal hairs, it generally will not reverse the terminalization of hairs.

Currently Available Lasers and Light Sources Used for Hair Removal

In the USA, the Food and Drug Administration (FDA) has traditionally used electrolysis results as a benchmark to evaluate laser treatment efficacy, despite the near lack of significant scientific data about electrolysis. In the initially submitted studies, all hair removal devices were required to show a 30% decrease in hair growth at 3 months after a single treatment (Tope et al. 1998).

This criterion clearly does not equate with permanent hair loss, as a delay in hair growth, which usually lasts for 1–3 months, is simply consistent with the induction of the telogen stage. Permanent hair reduction results should be based on the cyclic growth phases for hair follicles, and should refer to a significant reduction in the number of terminal hairs after a given treatment. There must be a reduction that is stable for a period of time longer than the complete growth cycle of hair follicles at any given body site.

Multiple laser systems are currently available and approved by the FDA for hair removal. The lists below include the more popular systems. They are not meant to be all-inclusive.

Ruby Lasers

Ruby lasers (694 nm), used for hair removal includes:
- Epilaser/E2000 (Palomar, Lexington, MA)
- EpiPulse Ruby (Lumenis, Santa Clara, CA)
- RubyStar (Aesculap Meditec., Irvine, CA)

Epilaser/E2000 (Palomar). With this laser, light is delivered through a fiber, and two different spot sizes (10 mm and 20 mm) are available. A retroreflector is built into the hand piece, allowing photon recycling and therefore higher energy delivery (Anderson et al. 1999; Ross et al. 1996). Depending on skin type or hair thickness, a single pulse of 3 ms or twin pulses (i. e., two 3-ms pulses delivered with a delay of 100 ms) can be chosen. The E2000 uses a sapphire-cooled handpiece (Epiwand) to protect the epidermis during laser irradiation. The sapphire lens is actively cooled to 0° or –10°C and put in direct contact with the skin.

The long-pulsed EpiPulse Ruby laser (Lumenis) employs triple-pulse technology with 10-ms intervals between pulses. This train of pulses keeps the follicle temperature sufficiently high to cause destruction. Epidermal cooling is achieved by applying a thick layer of cooled transparent gel on the skin.

The RubyStar (Aesculap-Meditec) is a dual-mode ruby laser that uses a contact skin cooling method. It can operate in the nanosecond Q-switched mode for the treatment of tattoos and pigmented lesions and in the normal millisecond mode for hair removal. Its integrated cooling device consists of a cooled contact handpiece which precools the skin before laser pulse delivery.

Although the mechanism of ruby laser induction of follicular injury is likely to be thermal, the precise contributions of photomechanical damage or thermal denaturation to follicular injury are unknown. It is possible that after absorption of radiant energy, the large temperature differences between the absorbing melanosomes and their surroundings produce a localized rapid volume expansion. This would then lead to microvaporization or "shock waves," which cause structural damage to the hairs (Anderson et al. 1983). On the other hand, thermal denaturation leading to melanosomal damage is also possible. Histologic evaluation of laser-treated mouse skin has revealed evidence of thermal coagulation and asymmetric focal rupture of the follicular epithelium (Lin et al. 1998). Secondary damage to adjacent organelles could theoretically result either from thermal diffusion or from propagation of shock waves.

Because of its comparatively short ruby laser wavelength, this hair removal system is best suited for the treatment of dark hair in light skin. It also may be more efficacious than longer wavelength devices for the treatment of light hair or red to red-brown hair (Ross et al.

1999). Because of the high melanin absorption coefficient at 694 nm, the ruby laser must be used with caution in darkly pigmented or tan patients.

A number of reports have documented the efficacy of ruby laser hair removal in varying types of skin using different laser parameters. The published hair reduction rates have ranged from a 37% to 72% reduction 3 months after one to three treatments to a 38%–49% hair reduction 1 year after three treatment sessions (Williams et al. 1998). As would be expected, multiple treatments at 3- to 5-week intervals produce a greater degree of hair reduction than is seen after a single session. In general, higher delivered fluences do lead to better hair removal success, although complications also increase.

Studies with larger numbers of patients have confirmed that hair counts are reduced by approximately 30% after a single treatment with ruby laser (Williams et al. 1998). The effects of multiple treatments sessions are additive, as hair counts are reduced by approximately 60% after three or four treatment sessions. Whether 100% permanent hair removal can be achieved remains open to debate.

Alexandrite Lasers

Several long-pulsed alexandrite lasers (755 nm) are being used for hair removal, including:

- Apogee series (Cynosure, Chelmsford, MA)
- Epitouch ALEX (Lumenis, Santa Clara, CA)
- GentleLase (Candela, Wayland, MA)

The Apogee system (Cynosure) provides pulse durations between 5 and 40 ms and fluences up to 50 J/cm². A cooling handpiece (SmartCool) blows a continuous flow of chilled air into the treatment area. The scanner option (SmartScan) enables treatment of large areas with an unobstructed view, speedy treatment, and ease of use with minimal operator fatigue.

The Epitouch ALEX (Lumenis) delivers a 2-ms pulse duration, spot sizes of 5–10 mm, and fluences of 10–25 J/cm². A cooling gel is applied to the skin before treatment, and a scanning device can be used to treat larger body-surface areas.

The GentleLase (Candela) delivers a 3-ms pulse duration, spot sizes of 8–18 mm, and fluences ranging from 10 to 100 J/cm². It employs a dynamic cooling device (DCD) to protect the epidermis. The DCD cooling method uses short (5–100 ms) cryogen spurts, delivered to the skin surface through an electronically controlled solenoid valve; the quantity of cryogen delivered is proportional to the spurt duration.

There are a number of advantages in using long-pulsed alexandrite lasers for hair removal. Some of the long-pulsed alexandrite laser systems are compact and can be used in small rooms if adequate ventilation is available. Their flexible fiberoptic arm is easy to manipulate and provides access to hard-to-reach body areas. The large spot sizes and frequency (1–5 Hz) improves the possibility of rapidly treating large body areas.

The alexandrite laser wave length of 755 nm is absorbed about 20% less strongly by melanin compared with the ruby laser wavelength of 694 nm. Its absorption by the competing chromophore, oxyhemoglobin, is substantially increased as compared to the 694-nm wavelength. However, the longer wavelength of 755 nm penetrates more deeply into the dermis and is less absorbed by epidermal melanin. This theoretically decreases the risk of epidermal damage, especially in individuals with darker skin types.

Because dermal scattering decreases with increasingly longer wavelengths, 755-nm light penetrates deeper into tissue than does shorter wavelengths. In theory, the use of longer wavelengths should increase the ratio of energy deposited in the dermis relative to the epidermis. This would result in relatively increased bulb heating while at the same time promoting epidermal sparing (Ross et al. 1999).

The reported hair removal success rate using an alexandrite laser has ranged from 40% to 80% at 6 months after several treatments (Gorgu et al. 2000) In a controlled randomized study using a single 20 J/cm², 5- to 20-ms alexandrite laser on various anatomic sites, investigators reported a 40% reduction in hair growth 6 months after treatment. This increased to >50% (on the upper lip) if a second treatment was performed after 8 weeks. In another study, one treatment with a variable pulsed alexandrite laser produced maximum hair growth reduction at 6 months of 40%–56% for the lip, leg, and back. Finally, one study has noted a mean 74% bikini hair reduction 1 year after five alexandrite laser treatments.

Diode Lasers

Diode lasers (800 nm) used for hair removal include:
- LightSheer (Lumenis, Santa Clara, CA)
- Apex-800, (Iriderm, Mountain View, CA)
- LaserLite, (Diomed, Boston, MA)
- SLP 1000 (Palomar Medical Technologies, Lexington, MA)
- MeDioStar (Aesculap-Meditec, Irvine, CA)
- EpiStar (Nidek, Freemont, CA)

Although the myriad diode lasers vary in their delivered energies, spot sizes, pulse duration, and associated cooling devices, they all set a popular standard for efficiency, reliability, and portability.

Because of reduced scattering at the longer 810-nm diode wavelengths, light from the diode laser penetrates more deeply into the skin. At 800 nm, 24% of incident fluence reaches a depth of 3 mm, whereas only 5% reaches the same depth with 700-nm light (Ross et al. 1999). Also, 800-nm energy is 30% less absorbed by melanin than that of the ruby laser, yet the 800-nm wavelength leads to better optical penetration.

In general, the diode laser system has been found to be better tolerated by patients with darker skin types (V–VI) as compared to the ruby laser (Adrian et al. 2000). This is likely due to its longer wavelength, longer pulse width, and associated active cooling.

In a prospective controlled trial, the 810-nm diode laser demonstrated a significant reduction in hair growth (Lou et al. 2000). Overall, clinical studies with the diode laser system have reported variable success rates ranging from 65–75% hair reduction at 3 months after one to two treatments with fluences of 10–40 J/cm². This was increased to >75% hair reduction in 91% of subjects 8 months after three to four treatments at 40 J/cm² (Williams et al. 1999). As

expected, repeated treatments, generally at 4-week intervals, appears to improve results (Lou et al. 2000).

Nd:YAG Lasers

Millisecond Nd:YAG lasers (1064 nm) used for hair removal include:
- Lyra (Laserscope, San Jose, CA)
- CoolGlide (Cutera, Brisbane, CA)
- Yaglase (Depilase, Irvine, CA)
- Image (Sciton, Palo Alto, CA)
- VascuLight (Lumenis, Santa Clara, CA)

The longer Nd:YAG laser wavelength provides deeper penetration, a necessary factor in the attempt to achieve optimal laser hair removal results. In addition, the 1064-nm wavelength is relatively less absorbed by epidermal melanin than are the 694- to 810-nm wavelengths. It is this decreased melanin absorption that leads to the greater pigmented epidermal safety seen with these systems.

Although the 1064-nm wavelength is less well absorbed by melanin than shorter wavelengths, the absorption appears to be enough to achieve the selective photothermolysis of the pigmented hair follicle (Lin et al. 1998). The use of appropriate fluences and effective epidermal cooling devices leads to an effective hair removal device with little risk of complications when such lasers are used correctly. Although the relatively low melanin absorption would appear to be a disadvantage in the treatment of pigmented hair, the Nd:YAG laser's advantage is its ability to reduce the thermal damage of the laser-treated melanin containing epidermis. Thus, side effects are decreased in darker-skinned patients).

Although Nd:YAG laser treatment usually leads to less dramatic results when compared to other laser systems available for hair reduction, its 1064-nm wavelength decreased absorption by melanin may also cause a lesser incidence of epidermal side effects, including blistering and abnormal pigmentation (Nanni et al. 1999). Short-term hair reduction in the range of 20%–60% has been obtained with the long pulsed Nd:YAG lasers.

Early clinical studies have demonstrated less hair reduction/laser session with Nd:YAG lasers as compared to the published results with either ruby or alexandrite lasers

However, preliminary studies suggest that newer, high powered long-pulsed Nd:YAG lasers may provide hair loss comparable to that seen with other devices. The long-term efficacy and precise role of the long-pulsed Nd:YAG lasers remains to be established.

Q-Switched Nd:YAG Laser

Q-switched Nd:YAG lasers have been used to target topically applied carbon particles that have previously been applied to the hair follicle. This method was one of the first available laser hair removal techniques. This short term hair removal technique has also been used without the prior application of carbon.

Immediately after Q-switched 1064-nm laser irradiation of carbon coated hairs, the carbon is heated to its vaporization temperature of about 3,700 °C. Vaporization leads to a huge volume expansion with resultant supersonic proliferation of high pressure waves. These shock waves, in turn, produce mechanical damage, as well as the development of heat. It is not clear how much mechanical and/or heat energy produced by this mechanism is required for destruction of a hair follicle. However, histologic evidence of follicular damage is seen after such a laser exposure. This results in a clinical delay of hair growth.

Depending on the position and amount of the topically applied chromophore, as well as the energy administered, it may be possible to occasionally irreversibly damage a hair follicle even with a Q-switched laser.

Histologic studies have documented the presence of carbon in the follicle after low fluence Nd:YAG lasing. This carbon appears to penetrate superficially in a large number of follicles with and without a hair shaft in place; deep follicular penetration is rare. The disadvantages of this technique, therefore, appear to relate to the fact that that the carbon granules may not consistently reach the requisite hair bulge or bulb.

Different studies have compared the effectiveness of Q-switched Nd:YAG laser hair removal with ruby and alexandrite laser treatments. Millisecond pulse ruby and alexandrite lasers showed greater hair reduction than was seen with Q-switched Nd:YAG lasers. Relatively weak absorption by the innate target chromophore melanin of Q-switched Nd:YAG laser energy translates into less energy available to damage the follicle. Therefore, a lesser hair removal effect is seen.

Several studies have examined the 1064-nm Q-switched Nd:YAG laser with and without a topically applied chromophore. However, in one controlled study (Nanni et al. 1997), using a single Q-switched Nd:YAG laser treatment, 100% hair regrowth was observed at 6 months irrespective of the treatment. Although capable of inducing delayed regrowth, Q-switched Nd:YAG laser treatment appears to be ineffective at producing long-term hair removal.

Intense Pulsed Light Systems

Intense pulsed light (IPL) systems are high intensity pulsed light sources which emit polychromatic light in a broad wavelength spectrum of 515–1200 nm. The emitted wavelengths determine not only the absorption pattern of the emitted light but also the penetration depth of the light. With the aid of different cut-off filters (515–755 nm), which only allow a defined wavelength emission spectrum, the optimal wavelength spectrum can be filtered to correspond to the depth of the target structure (i. e., hair follicles). Similarly, the emitted wavelengths can be adopted to the patient's individual skin type. Higher cutoff filters reduce the emission of melanin-absorbing wavelengths; thus being safer for darker skin types.

The pulse duration of IPL systems can be set to a wide range of parameters. The use of single pulses is possible. In the alternative, high fluences can be divided into multiple pulses. The intervals between individual pulses can be set at values between 1 and 300 ms. This delay, in theory, allows the epidermis and smaller vessels to cool down between pulses while the heat is retained in the larger target (hair follicles). This

4

results in selective thermal damage. The extent of maximum delivered fluences and the spot size vary, depending on utilized IPL.

When an IPL is used, a transparent refrigerated gel is placed on the skin to cool the epidermis and to improve light delivery to the skin during treatment. The large rectangular spot sizes associated with most IPL hand pieces allows a large number of hairs to be treated simultaneously.

The IPL delivery of a broad range of wavelengths has some advantages. The presence of longer wavelengths provides better penetration depth into the dermis, while shorter wavelengths can be filtered out to protect the epidermis in darker-skinned individuals. Shorter emitted wavelengths may also be useful to treat red-brown hair (Ross et al. 1999).

One of the greatest technical advantages of IPL systems is the large exposure area that is used. This improves the resultant damage of deep follicles. A disadvantage is that the rectangular spot size prevents treatment of hair-bearing areas on marked convexities or concavities (Ross et al. 1999).

Several studies have demonstrated the long-term efficacy of IPL hair removal devices (Gold et al. 1997; Weiss et al. 1999). In one study of 67 subjects of Fitzpatrick skin phototypes I-IV, mean hair loss was 48% at 6 months or more after a single treatment. In another study, after a single treatment, hair reduction ranging from 33% to 60% was observed at 6 months after treatment. Further studies of 14 subjects treated with this technology and followed for >12 months after their last treatment showed a mean of 83% hair reduction was obtained after two to six treatments. As would be expected, repeated treatments appear to improve outcome. Despite this, some have suggested that more than three IPL treatments do not appear to increase the success rate. Not all would agree with this. Finally, treatment with IPL, with and without bipolar radiofrequency, has been said to be useful for the treatment of light-colored hair. Generally, more treatments are required and the results are not expected to be as good as those seen when treating darker-colored hairs.

Advantages

Laser-assisted hair removal is now an accepted successful treatment for the removal of unwanted hair. It has been proven to be more effective than electrolysis and clearly represents the best method for removing large areas of hair in a relatively short period of time.

Disadvantages

The theoretical explanations behind laser-assisted hair removal seem logical. However, questions do remain. It is very difficult to predict the ideal patient and ideal treatment parameters for each patient. Even the same patient may respond differently to the same parameters on two different treatment sessions.

It is impossible to estimate the exact amount of energy absorbed by each hair follicle after laser irradiation owing to skin nonhomogeneity, multilayering, and anisotrophic physical properties of hair growing at different angles in relation to the laser impact. In addition, because growing hair depths vary between 2 and 7 mm depending on the body location, laser absorption characteristics will vary depending on the anatomic site. Finally, the percentage of anagen and telogen hairs varies from site to site, from person to person, and from season to season. It is not even clear whether the treatment of anagen as compared to catagen or telogen hairs even matters.

Many studies now show the hair follicle to be an incredibly resilient structure, regrowing after a seemingly lethal injury. It is the delivery of adequate fluences, optimizing wavelengths, and pulse durations, while reducing unwanted epidermal injuries that leads to the optimal treatments of pigmented hair. Unfortunately, the treatment of unwanted light or white hairs remains a challenge.

Indications

Individuals may seek laser hair removal because of excess hair induced by genetics or associated medical conditions. More commonly, laser hair removal patients simply have unwanted hair that would be considered normal in distribution and density. Yet, these individuals for emotional, social, cultural, cosmetic, or other reasons want the hair to be removed. Also, individuals with pseudofolliculitis barbae, a relatively common disorder seen with coarse, curly hairs that occurs in glabrous skin, often seek laser hair removal.

The ideal candidate for laser hair removal is a dark-haired, fair-skinned individual with little melanin within the overlying epidermis. Such patients tolerate the use of more effective higher fluences and relatively shorter wavelengths. In darker-skinned individuals it may be preferable to utilize a longer wavelength laser device. Epidermal protection is also afforded by utilizing longer pulse durations and active cooling.

Contraindications

There are a number of relative contraindications that the laser physician should consider before treatment. The physician should ascertain that the patient has realistic expectations from the laser treatment. Patients with a history of hypertrophic or keloidal scarring should be treated more conservatively, using test spots and lower fluences. Likewise, patients with a history of recent isotretinoin use should be treated less aggressively.

Any patient with a history of herpes simplex infections should be given prophylactic antiviral therapy prior to any laser treatment at that anatomic site. Patients who regularly take aspirin or anticoagulant therapy should discontinue taking these medications at least 10 days prior to treatment, if possible. If these medications are not discontinued, patients may have more bruising, as these medications can predispose to vessel extravasation after treatment. It is recommended that patients having a history of persistent postinflammatory hyperpigmentation, darkly tanned skin, or skin types greater than Fitzpatrick phototype III, not be treated with lasers having shorter wavelengths, as such individuals are at a greater risk of postinflammatory hyperpigmentation.

Patients having photosensitivity disorders, or using systemic medications known to be photosensitizing, should be carefully screened.

Although laser treatment in itself is inherently safe in pregnancy, the treatment does cause pain and can be distressing, and is best deferred in some patients until after delivery.

All patients should be instructed to postoperatively avoid sun exposure and wear a broad spectrum sunscreen of SPF 30 or higher on treated exposed areas.

Consent

Informed consent is mandatory and should include treatment options, potential reasonable risks and benefits. One should avoid any guarantees. Figure 4.1 is a suggested consent for laser/light source hair removal.

Personal Laser Approach

Alexandrite Laser

Most individuals are no longer using ruby lasers. However, the same general approach to alexandrite laser treatments would apply if the ruby laser was used for hair removal in lighter skin types. We have found the alexandrite lasers to be very helpful in treating Fitzpatrick I–III skin phenotypes (Figs. 4.2–4.14). Although it has been suggested that alexandrite lasers, with their longer 755-nm wavelength, are safer in treating darker complexions than are ruby lasers, we have not consistently found this to be the case. It would appear that the ability to treat darker complexions with alexandrite lasers may be more related to the longer pulse durations emitted by some of these systems. It should be noted that unless appropriate cooling is utilized, some Fitzpatrick skin phenotype III and even sun-tanned type II complexioned individuals tend to have postinflammatory pigmentary changes after laser treatment.

OPERATIVE CONSENT: LASER/LIGHT SOURCE HAIR REMOVAL

Patient . . . .   Date . . . .

I am aware that laser/light source hair removal is a relatively new procedure. My doctor has explained to me that much of what has been written about these methods in newspapers, magazines, television, etc. has been sensationalized. I understand the nature, goals, limitations, and possible complications of this procedure, and I have discussed alternative forms of treatment. I have had the opportunity to ask questions about the procedure, its limitations and possible complications (see below).

I clearly understand and accept the following:
1. The goal of these surgeries, as in any cosmetic procedure, is improvement, not perfection.
2. The final result may not be apparent for months postoperatively.
3. In order to achieve the best possible result, more than one procedure will be required. There will be a charge for any further operations performed.
4. Strict adherence to the postoperative regimen (i.e., appropriate wound care and sun avoidance) is necessary in order to achieve the best possible result.
5. The surgical fee is paid for the operation itself and subsequent postoperative office visits. There is no guarantee that the expected or anticipated results will be achieved.

Although complications following laser/light source hair removal are infrequent, I understand that the following may occur:
1. Bleeding, which in rare instances could require hospitalization.
2. Infection is rare, but should it occur, treatment with antibiotics may be required.
3. Objectionable scarring is rare, but various kinds of scars are possible.
4. Alterations of skin pigmentation may occur in the areas of laser surgery. These are usually temporary, but rarely can be permanent.
5. A paradoxical increased hair growth may occur at or near treated sites. This generally responds to further treatments.

This authorization is given for the purpose of facilitating my care and shall supersede all previous authorizations and/or agreements executed by me. My signature certifies that I understand the goals, limitations and possible complications of laser surgery, and that I wish to proceed with the operation.

. . . .
Patient

. . . .
Witness   Date

Fig. 4.1. Consent form

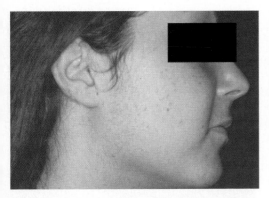

Fig. 4.2. Before alexandrite laser hair removal

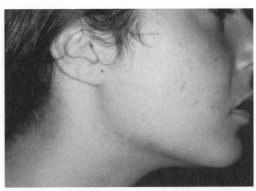

Fig. 4.3. Six months after five alexandrite hair removal sessions

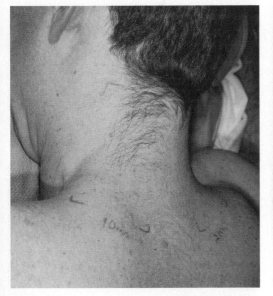

Fig. 4.4. Before alexandrite laser hair removal

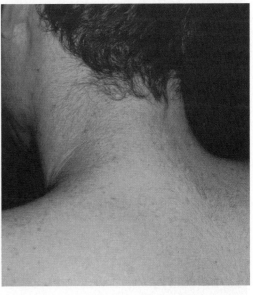

Fig. 4.5. Six months after five alexandrite hair removal sessions

Diode Laser

We have found the 810-nm diode lasers very useful in treating Fitzpatrick I–IV skin phenotypes (Figs. 4.15–4.18). The laser should always be used with a cooling device. When used with the longer emitted 30-ms pulse durations, some darker Fitzpatrick skin phenotypes can be treated with a lessening of postinflammatory pigmentary changes. Diode systems are small, portable and very user-friendly.

As a general rule, somewhat lower fluences are required for effective hair removal than are required with the ruby lasers. This may be related to the deeper penetration of the 800-nm wavelength.

Nd:YAG Laser

We have found the nanosecond Q-switched Nd:YAG lasers to be highly effective in inducing

4

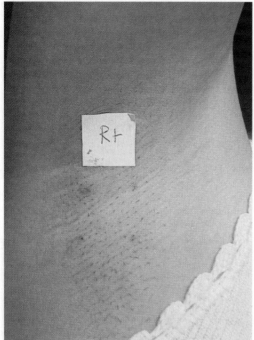

Fig. 4.6. Before alexandrite laser hair removal

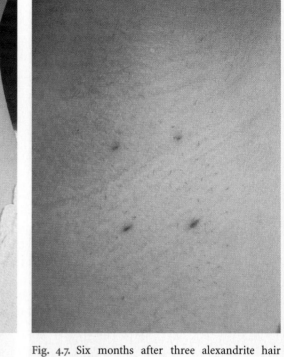

Fig. 4.7. Six months after three alexandrite hair removal sessions

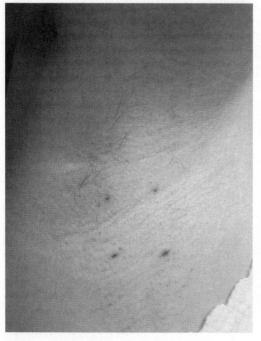

Fig. 4.8. Nine months after three alexandrite hair removal sessions

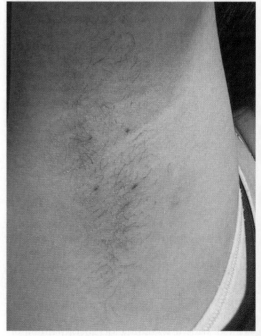

Fig. 4.9. Before alexandrite laser hair removal

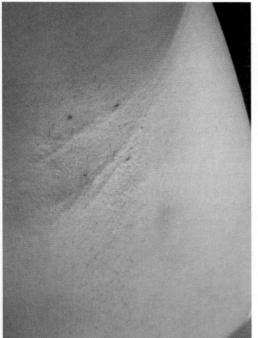

Fig. 4.10. Six months after three alexandrite hair removal sessions

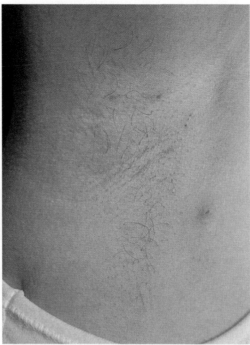

Fig. 4.11. Nine months after three alexandrite hair removal sessions

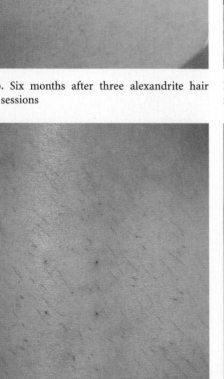

Fig. 4.12. Before alexandrite laser hair removal

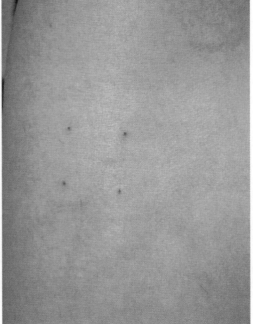

Fig. 4.13. Six months after three alexandrite hair removal sessions

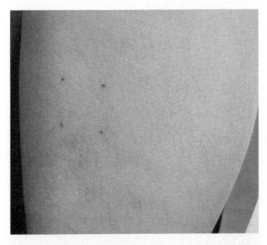

Fig. 4.14. Nine months after three alexandrite hair removal sessions

temporary short-term hair removal. Skin cooling is not required when a nanosecond laser is used. This contrasts with the requisite need for some form of epidermal cooling with virtually all millisecond hair removal lasers.

When the Q-switched Nd:YAG laser technique is utilized with a topical carbon suspension, there is often a greenish hue to the area being treated when visualized through goggles. This is presumably due to the interaction between the 1064-nm wavelength and the carbon chromophore. When the 1064-nm Q-switched Nd:YAG laser is used without topical carbon chromophore, dark terminal hairs often turn white on laser impact. Usually no post-

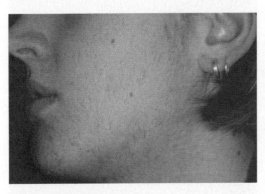

Fig. 4.15. Before diode laser hair removal

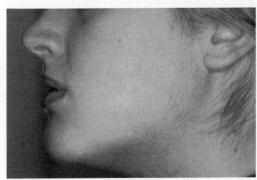

Fig. 4.16. Six months after two diode hair removal sessions

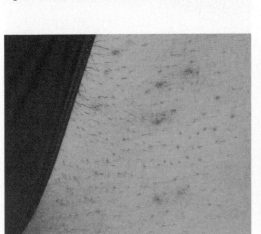

Fig. 4.17. Before diode laser hair removal

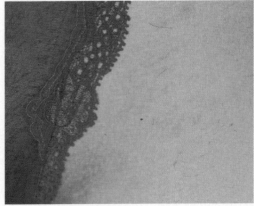

Fig. 4.18. Six months after five diode hair removal sessions

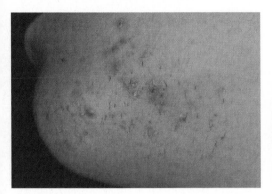

Fig. 4.19. Before Nd:YAG laser hair removal

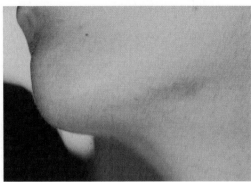

Fig. 4.20. Six months after five Nd:YAG laser hair removal sessions. Note not only decreased hair but also improvement in pseudofolliculitis barbae

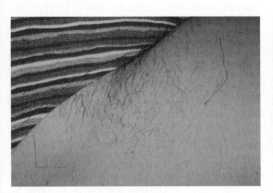

Fig. 4.21. Before IPL hair removal

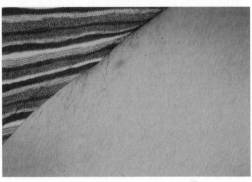

Fig. 4.22. Six months after three IPL hair removal sessions

treatment crusting is noted. Erythema may vary from nonexistent to significant in its extent. It is quite safe to treat individuals who have darker complexions with nanosecond Q-switched Nd:YAG laser.

Millisecond Nd:YAG laser systems are the safest laser hair removal systems for Fitzpatrick skin types V–VI (Figs. 4.19, 4.20). Although they can also be used for lighter skin types, we have not found the same degree of success when these lasers are compared to the shorter wavelength systems. Although postinflammatory pigmentary changes from this laser are rare, such changes can be occasionally expected in some individuals with dark complexions.

IPL

We have found intense pulsed light sources to be useful in treating Fitzpatrick I and IV skin phenotypes (Figs. 4.21–4.24). Although some IPL sources are FDA cleared in the USA for Fitzpatrick skin phenotypes V, we have found that the incidence of postinflammatory changes may be too high for practical use in some of these individuals. In choosing emitted pulse durations, we have noted that shorter pulse durations are more helpful for finer hairs, while longer pulse durations appear to have greater efficacy in treating thicker hairs. In addition, longer pulse durations, because of their epidermal pigment sparing capacity, are chosen for darker skin phenotypes. The choice of pulsing mode and inter-

4

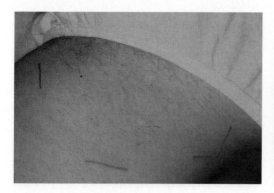

Fig. 4.23. Before IPL hair removal

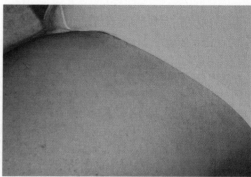

Fig. 4.24. Six months after three IPL hair removal sessions

pulse times are also dictated by complexion. Darker complexions are usually treated with a double/triple pulse and longer interpulse times, in comparison with the parameters chosen with lighter skin complexions. As is true for all lasers used for hair removal, the higher the fluences, the better the results. The fluence chosen should be as high as can be tolerated without creating an epidermal blister.

Intense pulsed light sources have shown the greatest safety when used with optimal skin cooling.

Treatment Approach

The hair removal treatment technique with all lasers and intense pulsed light sources commences with preoperative shaving of the treatment site. This reduces treatment-induced odor, prevents long pigmented hairs that lie on the skin surface from conducting thermal energy to the adjacent epidermis, and promotes transmission of laser energy down the hair follicle. A small amount of posttreatment crusting and erythema is to be expected. In darkly pigmented or heavily tanned individuals, it may be beneficial to use topical hydroquinones and meticulous sunscreen protection for several weeks prior to treatment in order to reduce inadvertent injury to epidermal pigment. Individuals with recent suntans should not be treated until pretreatment hydroquinones have been used for at least 1 month. Postinflamma-

tory pigmentary changes are still to be expected in individuals who have darker complexions.

All of the lasers and intense pulsed light sources described in this chapter, when used with almost all fluences, can lead to temporary hair loss at all treated areas. However, choosing appropriate anatomic locations and using higher fluences will increase the likelihood of permanent hair reduction after multiple treatments. Even though permanent hair loss is not to be expected in all individuals, lessening of hair density and thickness is an expected finding.

The ideal treatment parameters must be individualized for each patient, based on clinical experience and professional judgment. For individuals who have darker complexions, the novice might consider delivering the laser energy in several individual test pulses at an inconspicuous site with lower energy fluences. The delivered energies are then slowly increased. Undesirable epidermal changes such as whitening and blistering are to be avoided.

Prolonged and permanent hair loss may occur following the use of all the aforementioned described millisecond systems. However, great variation in treatment results is often seen. Most patients with brown or black hair obtain a 2- to 6-month growing delay after a single treatment. There is usually only mild discomfort at the time of treatment. Pain may be diminished by the use of topical or injected anesthetics.

Transient erythema and edema are also occasionally seen and irregular pigmentation of

1- to 3-months duration is often noted. These changes are far less common after treatment with an Nd:YAG laser. Permanent skin changes, depigmentation, or scarring is rare.

Finally, it is true for all hair removal lasers that the higher the delivered fluences, the better the results. The fluence chosen should be as high as can be tolerated without creating an epidermal blister.

Postoperative Considerations

The use of ice packs may reduce postoperative pain and minimize swelling. Analgesics are usually not required unless extensive areas are treated. Prophylactic courses of antiviral agents should be considered in patients with a history of herpes simplex infections in the to-be-treated area. Topical antibiotic ointment applied twice daily is indicated if posttreatment epidermal injury occurred. Mild topical steroid creams may be prescribed to reduce swelling and erythema. Any trauma, such as picking or scratching of the area, should be avoided. During the first week of healing, sun exposure should be avoided or sunblocks used. Make-up may be applied on the next day unless blistering or crusts have developed. The damaged hair is often shed during or after the first week of the treatment. Patients should be reassured that this not a sign of hair regrowth.

Complications

The incidence of cutaneous adverse effects after laser hair removal is both patient and laser parameter related. Patients with darker-colored skin, especially skin types V and VI, are more likely to experience cutaneous adverse effects, related to the abundance of melanin in their epidermis. However, such complications are not limited to patients with genetically determined dark skin. This may also be seen in patients with darker skin due to other reasons, such as sun-tanning and lentiginous photoaging. The incidence of adverse effects will be modified by utilized wavelength, fluence, pulse duration, and associated cooling.

Pigmentary Changes

There is a remarkable variation in the reported incidence of postoperative pigmentary changes after laser hair removal. Unfortunately most studies have not been carried out under standardized conditions. In different studies, varied laser parameters have been used, follow-up periods have varied from 90 days to 2 years, and the preoperative skin characteristics were not standardized (hair color, skin pigmentation, anatomical region). Finally, the majority of studies estimate the incidence of side effects by subjective clinical evaluation.

In general, laser-induced pigmentary changes depend on the degree of preoperative pigmentation. Lighter skin types potentially experience more postoperative hyperpigmentation. Darker skin types experience more sub-clinical hypopigmentation. This finding is in accordance with the fact that laser light in dark-skinned types is strongly absorbed by the epidermal melanin, leading to potential melanocytic damage (Anderson 1994). Conversely, thermal effects in lighter skin may provoke postinflammatory hyperpigmentation.

Hypopigmentation

Transient posttreatment hypopigmentation occurs in 10%–17% of patients (Grossman et al. 1996; Bjerring et al. 1998; Williams et al. 1998). The exact etiology of postlaser hair removal-induced hypopigmentation is unclear, but may be related to the destruction of melanocytes, suppression of melanogenesis, or the redistribution of melanin in the keratinocytes.

Hyperpigmentation

Transient posttreatment hyperpigmentation occurs in 14%–25% of patients (Grossman et al. 1996; Bjerring et al. 1998; Williams et al. 1998), and is normally related to melanocytic-induced stimulation. The causes of this hyperpigmentation include delayed tanning, epidermal injury, or an immediate pigment darkening phenomenon resulting from photo-oxidation of

4

pre-existing melanin. The darkening is usually transient, lasting only 3–4 weeks and resolves without sequelae in most individuals (McDaniel 1993).

A potentially more serious hyperpigmentation resulting from epidermolysis and blistering can occur at energy thresholds higher than those associated with immediate pigment darkening. This can be associated with permanent dyschromia.

Pain

Laser and light source heat-induced destruction of hair follicles is not pain free, as the hair follicle is well endowed with pain fibers arranged in a well-organized neovascular bundle. The intensity of pain varies with the delivered fluence, utilized wave length, pulse duration, spot size, repetition rate, laser interpulse spacing, and skin pigmentation. Regional body areas such as the lip and groin, and chronically sun-exposed and tanned areas, also have been associated with greater amounts of pain perception. In addition, with increasing pulse duration, heat diffusion is likely to raise the temperature around the follicle and increase the level of pain. Finally, pain can be perceived differently at different times of the month. During menstruation, the skin appears to be more sensitive to pain and laser hair removal can be more uncomfortable.

Scarring and Textural Changes

Despite the presence of severe macroscopic cutaneous damage, collagen and elastin networks in the dermis are found to be normal in the majority of the laser hair removal-treated patients. Scarring can occur, but is rare.

Effects on Tattoos and Freckles

Lightening of tattoos and loss of freckles or pigmented lesions after laser-assisted hair removal are common. Patients should be made aware of this possibility.

Infections

Herpes simplex infections are uncommon after laser and light source treatment of hair removal, but may occur, especially in patients with strong prior history of outbreaks. Eruptions most commonly are seen on or around the lip. Although the risk of bacterial infection is extremely low, it may occur if there is laser-induced epidermal damage.

Plume

The plume generated by the vaporized hair shaft has a sulphur smell and in large quantities can be irritating to the respiratory tract. A smoke evacuator is advised.

The Future

The incredible amount of attention attracted by laser and light source hair removal techniques reflects a demand for more practical, tolerable, effective, and safer epilation techniques. At this time, effective light and white hair removal techniques do not exist. Research into techniques that light activate hair may be a part of the future treatment of nonpigmented hairs.

References

Adrian RM, Shay KP (2000) 800 nanometer diode laser hair removal in African American patients: a clinical and histologic study. J Cutan Laser Ther 2: 183–190

Altshuler GB, Anderson RR, Smirnove MZ, et al (2001) Extended theory of selective photothermolysis. Lasers Surg Med 29:416–432

Anderson RR (1994) Laser-tissue interactions. In: Baxter SH (ed) Cutaneous laser surgery. The art and science of selective photothermolysis. Mosby, St Louis, p 1–19

Anderson RR, Parrish JA (1983) Selective photothermolysis: Precise microsurgery by selective absorption of pulsed radiation. Science 220:524–527

Anderson RR, Dierickx CC, Altshuler GB, et al (1999) Photon recycling. A new method of enhancing hair removal Lasers Surg Med 11 Suppl:190

Bjerring P, Zachariae H, Lybecker H, et al (1998) Evaluation of free-running ruby laser for hair removal Acta Derm Venereol 78:48–51

Gold MH, Bell MW, Foster TD, et al (1997) Long-term epilation using the EpiLight broad band, intense-pulsed light hair removal system. Dermatol Surg 23:909–913

Gorgu M, Aslan G, Akoz T, et al (2000) Comparison of alexandrite laser and electrolysis for hair removal Dermatol Surg 26:37–41

Grossman MC, Dierickx CC, Farnelli W, et al (1996) Damage to hair follicles by normal-mode ruby laser pulses. J Am Acad Dermatol 35:889–894

Lin TD, Manuskiatti W, Dierickx CC, et al (1998) Hair growth cycle affects hair follicle destruction by ruby laser pulses. J Invest Dermatol 111:107–113

Lou WW, Quintana AT, Geranemus RG, et al (2000) Prospective study of hair reduction by diode laser (800 nm) with long-term follow-up. Dermatol Surg 26:428–432

McDaniel DH (1993) Clinical usefulness of the hexascan. J Dermatol Surg Oncol 19:312

Nanni CA, Alster TS (1997) Optimizing treatment parameters for hair removal using a topical carbon-based solution and 1064 nm Q-switched neodymium:YAG laser energy. Arch Dermatol 133:1546–1549

Nanni CA, Alster TS (1999) Laser-assisted hair removal: side effects of Q-switched Nd:YAG, long-pulsed ruby, and alexandrite lasers. J Am Acad Dermatol 41:165–171

Ohshiro T, Maruyama Y (1983) The ruby and argon lasers in the treatment of nevi. Ann Acad Med Singapore 12(2):388

Ross EV, Rathyen JS, Gandet T, et al (1996) Recycling wasted photons: A device to increase laser energy used in surgery. Lasers Surg Med 8(Suppl):87

Ross EV, Ladin Z, Kreidel M, et al (1999) Theoretical considerations in laser hair removal Dermatol Clin 17:333–355

Tope WD, Hordinsky MK (1998) A hair's breath closer? Arch Dermatol 134:867–869

Weiss RA, Weiss MA, Marwaha S, et al (1999) Hair removal with a noncoherent filtered flashlamp intense-pulsed light source. Lasers Surg Med 24:128–132

Wheeland RG (1997) Laser-assisted hair removal Dermatol Clin 15(3):469–477

Williams R, Havoonjian H, Isagholian K, et al (1998) A clinical study of hair removal using the long-pulsed ruby laser. Dermatol Surg 24:837–842

Williams RM, Gladstone HB, Moy RL (1999) Hair removal using an 810 nm gallium aluminum arsenide semiconductor diode laser: a preliminary study. Dermatol Surg 25:935–937

Zenzie HH, Altshuler GB, Anderson RR, et al (2000) Evaluation of cooling for laser dermatology. Lasers Surg Med 26:130–144

Ablative and Nonablative Facial Resurfacing

Suzanne L. Kilmer, Natalie Semchyshyn

5

Core Messages

- Ablative and non-ablative laser resurfacing lead to an improvement in photodamaged skin.
- Ablative laser resurfacing produces a significant wound, but long-lasting clinical results.
- Nonablative resurfacing is cosmetically elegant, but generally only leads to subtle results.
- Visible light nonablative devices lead to a lessening of erythema and superficial pigmentary skin changes
- Midinfrared infrared laser devices promote better skin quality and skin toning.
- The role of newer plasmakinetic and fractional resurfacing devices has yet to be determined.

History

Ablative resurfacing was first introduced in the mid 1990s. Technological advancements with carbon dioxide (CO_2) lasers had emerged to minimize their thermal impact on tissue and, subsequently, possible clinical uses were explored. Two types of CO_2 lasers were developed. The first utilized ultrashort pulse durations to minimize heat deposition in the tissue. The other utilized the laser beam in a continuous wave (CW) mode, in conjunction with a scanning device, to shorten the laser dwell time and, thereby, minimize thermal damage (Lask et al. 1995). These lasers were first used for the treatment of rhytides and acne scars; however, investigators soon discovered that superficial

sun damage changes, including lentigines, as well as actinic keratoses, fine lines, and other superficial imperfections also improved. Additionally, the deposition of heat was noted to cause a tissue-tightening effect, which softened deeper wrinkles (Fitzpatrick et al. 2000). The CO_2 laser proved to be very effective; however, as the technology expanded into the dermatologic and plastic surgeon's armamentarium, it was found to have significant side effects, especially in inexperienced hands. Many patients experienced erythema that lasted for weeks to months as well as temporary hyperpigmentation, acne, and contact sensitivity to topical products. Yeast, bacterial, and viral infections were a potential problem. Prolonged hypopigmentation and scarring, although infrequent, were also of great concern.

In an effort to decrease the risk/side effect profile, the use of erbium lasers was explored (Zachary 2000) These short-pulsed lasers, with stronger water absorption at 2.94 µm were less injurious to deeper tissues; they ablated tissue but left little residual thermal damage. Unfortunately it became apparent that this laser, although good for smoothing out the surface, did not lead to the same tightening effect as was noted with the CO_2 lasers. The next level of advancement entailed increasing the pulse width of the erbium lasers to include some deposition of heat, which would allow tightening (Pozner and Goldberg 2000). In addition, lasers were developed that combined both erbium and CO_2 lasers to allow heat deposition by the CO_2 component as well as pure ablation by the erbium component. The potential benefit was great; however, side effects continued to be present (Tanzi and Alster 2003). A recent paper showed that utilizing a topical anesthetic, which hydrated the skin, minimized side effects even with pure CO_2 lasers. In this study, a decreased incidence of prolonged erythema, pigmentary changes, and scarring were noted (Kilmer 2003).

Despite these advances, the significant amount of downtime associated with ablative resurfacing has led to the development of nonablative lasers to improve solar damage, including rhytides, telangiectases, and pigmentation. Nonablative technology evolved beginning with the use of early-pulsed dye lasers (Zelickson 1999) It had been noted that using the pulsed dye laser for the treatment of port wine stains that had been scarred from previous argon laser treatment improved not only the port wine stain, but the scars as well. In addition, patients with facial telangiectasies or poikiloderma of Civatte commented on their improved appearance.

These early studies showed that the pulsed dye laser not only improved rhytides but also caused histological changes in the dermis consistent with improvement of sun-damaged collagen. Similarly, the Q-switched Nd:YAG laser used in combination with a topical carbon suspension for laser hair removal was noted to diminish fine lines, most likely due to a photomechanical effect. Lasers with an affinity for water absorption were then investigated for their effects on wrinkle improvement. These lasers, which include the 1320-nm and 1450-nm systems, deliver heat into the dermis to trigger a wound-healing response. In these cases, epidermal damage was avoided by a concomitant cooling mechanism. Laser-induced histological changes showed increased fibroblast activity and new collagen deposition. These changes were similar to those seen with both the pulse dye and Q-switched Nd:YAG lasers. Over time, there has been an ever-increasing surge in patients demanding a "no downtime" wrinkle treatment and, consequently, the field of nonablative facial rejuvenation has expanded tremendously. Because ablative and nonablative lasers and their indications, benefits, risks, and treatment techniques vary so greatly they are separated in the discussion below. Ablative laser resurfacing will be discussed first, followed by the various nonablative technologies.

Ablative Resurfacing

Currently Available Technology

After a decade of ablative resurfacing, the mainstays remain both the CO_2 and erbium lasers. As noted above, the CO_2 lasers are available in one of two forms: the ultrashort pulsed and the rapidly scanned versions. The UltraPulse is the oldest and most well known of the pulsed versions. The SilkTouch and FeatherTouch were the more popular of the scanned versions. The TruePulse had an ultrashort pulse width and caused the least thermal damage of any CO_2 lasers.

The available erbium lasers include short-pulse and variable-pulsed lasers (with a pulse range typically in the microsecond to 10-ms range). Increasing the pulse width correlates directly with an increase in residual thermal damage, providing possible additional benefit as well as potential side effects. Of note, however, the short-pulse erbium lasers are not risk-free. Since the ablation depth of injury is an important factor, and erbium lasers can ablate to significant depths, the risk of scarring can be significant if these lasers are used incorrectly.

Advantages

Ablative resurfacing's biggest advantage is its efficacy. With one procedure, a significant reduction in wrinkles, solar lentigines, keratoses, surface irregularities, and skin laxity is noted. Five to ten years can be removed from a person's perceived age. The effect is immediate, in contrast to nonablative methods where results improve slowly over time. The effect is also predictable and, in most cases, at least 50% improvement is noted.

Most epidermal irregularities can be removed with a single pass. Subsequent passes allow for more tightening or further sculpting. The improvement in pigmentary changes, superficial growths, scars, fine lines, and skin laxity is dramatic. Skin tones are evened out and returned to normal nonsun-exposed color. Often, pores are diminished and solar elastotic changes are removed. Nevi, sebaceous hyperplasia, and other dermal tumors can be flattened. Actinic keratoses are removed and any superficial basal cell carcinomas (BCC) can be treated at the same session. In fact, several patients with a long history of BCCs occurring on both facial and body areas have not experienced new tumors on the face subsequent to CO_2 facial resurfacing – even though they continue to produce tumors on their nonfacial areas (S.L. Kilmer, personal observation).

Disadvantages

The disadvantage of ablative resurfacing is the significant downtime required during the recovery period. During the first week, erythema and edema are significant, wound care is necessary, and social activities come to a halt. Postoperative edema decreases after the first 3–4 days, whereas the erythema is prominent for the first week until re-epithelialization occurs and slowly diminishes over the next few weeks. The risk of infection, pigmentary changes and scarring is higher in the immediate postoperative period, as it is in any procedure where de-epithelialization occurs. Makeup is necessary for several weeks to months until any residual erythema and postinflammatory hyperpigmentation diminishes. Contact dermatitis may be more easily triggered in the postlaser disrupted epidermis, leading to pruritis and erythema. Acne, activated by the occlusive effect of the petrolatum or other dressings, is more common in the treated area and may take several weeks to clear. Relative hypopigmentation can be seen as removal of the acquired sun damage or "actinic bronzing" returns the skin to its normal nonsun-exposed color; this underscores the need for careful blending (feathering) into any surrounding areas of untreated sundamaged skin during the procedure. Of greater concern is the development of either permanent delayed hypopigmentation or scarring.

Indications

The most common indications for ablative resurfacing include wrinkles and acne scars. This procedure is especially helpful when pho-

todamage is a significant component as actinic keratoses and lentigines are easily ablated. Epidermal lesions such as seborrheic keratoses and even some dermal lesions such as sebaceous hyperplasia, nevi, trichoepitheliomas, and syringomas can be smoothed out. Superficial basal cell carcinomas can be treated with CO_2 laser resurfacing in a manner similar to desiccation and curettage. It appears that this modality also decreases the risk for the development of future actinic keratoses and basal cell carcinomas (S.L. Kilmer, personal observation).

Contraindications

There are few true contraindications. A personal or family history of vitiligo should be considered a relative contraindication. Theoretically, a Koebner phenomenon could occur and bring out vitiligo in the laser-treated areas. Scleroderma patients should be counseled that ablative resurfacing could exacerbate their disease, although reports of successful treatment exist (T. Alster, personal communication). Darker-skinned patients need to understand the likelihood of hyperpigmentation, which is usually temporary but may be long-lasting. The use of hydroquinone preparations with vitamin A derivatives, glycolic acid and/or topical corticosteroids, and good sunscreen minimized this problem. Patients with very fair and fine-pored skin appear to be at greatest risk for delayed hypopigmentation, which can be permanent. Unrealistic expectations and inability or unwillingness to perform wound care are contraindications for ablative skin resurfacing.

Consent

Informed consent is mandatory and should include treatment options, potential risks, and benefits. No guarantees should be made. A carefully written, detailed consent that explains the above is suggested (Fig. 5.1).

CO₂ & ERBIUM LASER RESURFACING PATIENT INFORMATION AND CONSENT
WHAT IS LASER SKIN RESURFACING?

The carbon dioxide (CO_2) laser has been used for more than 25 years for treating the skin. An intense beam of light is emitted, which heats and vaporizes skin tissue instantly. Recently developed Carbon Dioxide and Erbium Lasers are able to perform highly specific vaporization of tissue using powerfully focused light to precisely remove the layers of skin, vaporizing the ridges of scars and wrinkles and smoothing out the surface of the skin. In addition, the skin often tightens and collagen remodeling occurs with layers of new collagen replacing sun-damaged collagen. The CO_2 laser tightens the skin more while the erbium laser is used more for sculpting. We may use both of these lasers to maximize benefit depending on each individuals' needs.

BENEFITS
Laser resurfacing may significantly reduce facial wrinkle lines and acne scarring. The length of time these benefits will last is unknown. Sun spots and brown spots are often removed as well.

RISKS AND DISCOMFORTS
The most common side effects and complications are explained below.

ERYTHEMA (redness of skin)
The laser-treated areas have a distinctive redness which is much more vivid than the areas not treated. This redness generally will last one to four months beyond the time required to heal the skin surface (usually 7 to 10 days). This redness represents increased blood flow from healing as well as new growth of the superficial tissue and fades gradually week to week.

INFLAMMATION (swelling)
This is common and varies from person to person. Most patients swell moderately, but in some patients, swelling is severe. Your skin may feel tight in the initial weeks following treatment.

HYPERPIGMENTATION (increased skin color)
This is common in those with dark complexions, and almost always is temporary.
It responds to the use of hydroquinone, UVA protective sunscreens, and topical retinoids postoperatively.

HYPOPIGMENTATION (decreased skin color)
This has been uncommon and although is usually related to the depth of the peel, can occur for unknown reasons even when the procedure has been performed properly. In addition, removing sun damaged skin can return you to your natural lighter color similar to areas on your body that have not had long term sun exposure (i.e., underarms). Delayed hypopigmentation can occur months – years after the procedure is performed and can be permanent.

SCARRING OR KELOIDS
Scarring is not anticipated as a consequence of this procedure, but any procedure in which the surface of the skin is removed can heal with scarring. This usually occurs because of some secondary factor which interferes with healing, such as infection, irritation, scratching, or poor wound care. Scarring from infection, irritation or scratching, does blend and ordinarily disappears in a few months, but some scarring may be permanent if it occurs. Hypertrophic scars or keloids in susceptible people may suddenly appear. Most of these respond to injections or special creams. Some scarring could be permanent. **Notify your physician if you have ever used Accutane as this can increase your risk for scarring.**

ALLERGIC REACTIONS
Allergic reactions or irritations to some of the medications or creams may develop. An increased sensitivity to wind and sun may occur, but is temporary and clears as the skin heals.
If you have had a cold sore or herpes outbreak in or around the area to be treated, let us know as treatment can reactivate it.

DRUG SIDE EFFECTS
The drugs that **may** be administered can have the following general side effects:

Retin-A, Renova, (or other topical Vitamin A creams)
Sensitivity to sunlight, including sunlamps, mild skin irritation or dryness.

Melanex, Soloquin Forte, Lustra, (Hydroquinones or bleaching creams)
Mild skin irritation, itching, burning sensation.

Fig. 5.1. Informed consent for ablative resurfacing

Zovirax and Valtrex (antivirals)
Headaches, nausea

Keflex and Zithromax (antibiotics)
Dizziness, headache, nausea, rash

Diflucan (antiyeast)
Headache, nausea

Toradol, (nonsteroidal ant-inflammatory)
Actinic ulcers, bleeding, asthma

Vicodin, Maxidone, Darvocet, and Percocet (pain medication)
Lightheadedness, dizziness, sedation, nausea and vomiting.

Valium
Dizziness, lightheadedness, sedation, and respiratory depression

EXPLANATION OF THE PROCEDURE
A personal interview and clinical examination will be conducted to obtain relevant facts about your medical history, dermatologic history, and any medications you are currently taking or have taken in the recent past. Preoperative vitamin A and C creams may be started prior to the procedure. A sunscreen with UVB and UVA protection should be applied every morning. If you have a dark complexion, you may also need to apply a bleaching gel. You will begin taking an antiviral medication the night before or the morning of the procedure. On the day of the procedure, you will begin taking an antibiotic by mouth for a minimum of 5 days. A topical anesthetic cream will be applied for 2 hours before the procedure to decrease pain. Valium, Vicodin, Toradol or similar pain medication may be given as needed for pain. Injections to block the facial nerve endings may be performed just prior to the procedure. Please plan to have someone drive you home after the procedure.

AFTER CARE
An aftercare sheet will be given to you on your surgery day. You will be required to soak the treated area for 10 minutes, every few hours, using 1 teaspoon of vinegar (white) per 2 cups of water. Aquaphor or Vaseline is to be kept on your face continuously for 6 to 8 days. Any scabs should be gently soaked off. After soaking, pat the skin dry with a towel and apply more ointment over the treated area. Oozing of clear fluids, mild to moderate swelling, and a mild burning sensation may occur. Redness is expected for 1 to 2 weeks after the procedure and will fade gradually over 4 to 12 weeks.

NO GUARANTEES
It is possible that you may derive no benefits from the above-described procedure. While this procedure is effective in most cases, no guarantees can be made that a specific patient will benefit from treatment. Do not sign this form unless you have had a chance to ask questions and have received satisfactory answers to all of your questions.

WAIVER OF LIABILITY
All insurance companies, including Medicare, only pay for services that they determine to be 'reasonable' and necessary. If your insurance company determines that a particular service is not reasonable and necessary under their program standards, they will deny payment for that service. **I believe that your insurance, or Medicare, will deny payment for Laser Resurfacing, for the following reason: Insurances usually do not pay for cosmetic procedures.**

CONSENT
MY SIGNATURE INDICATES THE FOLLOWING: 1) I HAVE READ AND I UNDERSTAND THE INFORMATION OUTLINED ABOVE; 2) I HAVE DISCUSSED MY QUESTIONS WITH THE DOCTOR OR HER STAFF. 3) **I AM AWARE THAT PAYMENT IS DUE 2 WEEKS PRIOR TO MY SURGERY DATE. I AUTHORIZE THE RELEASE OF MY PHOTOGRAPHS.**

DATE . . . . NAME OF PATIENT . . . . SIGNATURE OF PATIENT . . . .

DATE . . . . NAME OF WITNESS . . . . SIGNATURE OF WITNESS. . . . .

DATE . . . . NAME OF PHYSICIAN . . . . SIGNATURE OF PHYSICIAN . . . .

Fig. 5.1. Informed consent for ablative resurfacing (continued)

5

Personal Laser Technique

A successful ablative resurfacing procedure begins with a thorough preoperative evaluation. This evaluation should pay careful attention to patient expectations, preoperative photographs, and counseling about the perioperative period. Medications are prescribed to minimize potential infection and include a prophylactic antibiotic (typically a first-generation cephalosporin), antiviral (acyclovir or valcyclovir), and antiyeast (fluconazole) medications. A nonsteroidal anti-inflammatory agent and an analgesic are also prescribed to control postoperative discomfort. Patients are educated as to what to expect during the healing period; appropriate wound care for the first week is reviewed. Preoperatively, patients apply topical anesthetic cream EMLA (eutectic mixture of lidocaine and prilocaine) with occlusion 2.5 h prior to the procedure time (Fig. 5.2). Forty-five minutes before the procedure, EMLA is reapplied with occlusion. The following medications are also provided by mouth: diazepam, hydrocodone or similar analgesic, and intramuscular ketorolac.

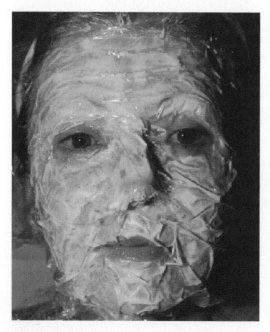

Fig. 5.2. EMLA with occlusion, preoperative

The first CO_2 ablative laser pass is performed mainly to remove the epidermis and feather peripherally to minimize any demarcation with surrounding nontreated skin. The second laser pass, and, if used, a third pass is for heat deposition to promote tightening. Finally, the erbium laser (in the ablation mode) can be used to remove superficial thermal necrosis for further sculpting of deeper rhytides and/or acne scars.

When the UltraPulse CO_2 laser specifically is used, the first pass is usually performed at a density of 7 for the main treatment areas. The previously described preoperative topical anesthetic technique leads to increased skin hydration and, consequently, allows the use of a higher density setting to more efficiently remove the epidermis. If no hydration is used, the first pass is performed at a density of 6. Hydration is mandatory, however, for treatment of the neck. When moving towards the jawline and hairline, the density is decreased to 6 and possibly 5 for higher risk patients. Progressing down the neck, density settings are decreased by one per row until the lowest setting of 1 is reached, allowing skip areas in the final row. The epidermis is then wiped free on the central face and other areas where a second pass is to be performed. The peripheral edges are usually left intact and the neck is never wiped.

The second CO_2 laser pass is performed at a density of 4–5 depending on the tightening needed and the risk for the area. The upper eyelids and the central face are typically treated at densities of 5, whereas mid cheeks and some lower eyelids may be treated with densities of 4. Delivered energies are also decreased towards the periphery. A second pass is rarely done on the lateral cheeks unless acne scarring is present. A third pass may be done on acne scars and in perioral and glabellar regions to deliver additional heat to enhance tightening. When using the EMLA topical anesthetic technique, the face is typically treated in sections (Fig. 5.3). All passes in a given area are performed before moving on to the next section.

In cases where deep rhytides or acne scars persist, the erbium laser in the ablative (shorter-pulsed) mode is helpful to sculpt the edges or to remove the superficial coagulative

Postoperative Care and Complications

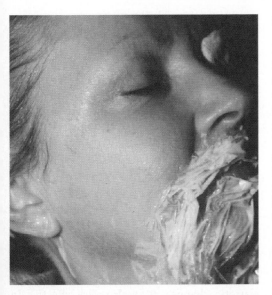

Both occlusive and nonocclusive types of dressings are available. Occlusive dressings entail a covering that occludes the skin and may provide more postoperative comfort. These are typically left in place for 1–3 days before removal followed by soaking of the treated area. The patient may then continue wound care with an open dressing. The downside to this method is that the occlusion can mask an infection and may, in fact, promote infection by harboring bacteria in the occluded area (Christian 2000). Open dressings are usually petrolatum-based ointments that provide an occlusive-like effect and allow for easy visualization and monitoring of the healing skin. Frequent soaking with dilute acetic acid promotes healing and inhibits bacterial growth. A variety of petrolatum-based products have been used. Regular vegetable oil-based shortening is also an excellent choice. It is the product with the least likelihood of triggering a topical allergic or irritant dermatitis. Vegetable oil-based shortening is usually not the first line product, because of its lack of elegance. However, if an allergic or irritant reaction occurs while using another open dressing, it is our first choice substitute.

Fig. 5.3. EMLA with occlusion; the face is treated with the CO_2 laser in sections, as shown

necrotic layer, which can hinder healing. The utilized erbium laser energy, and spot size, depends on the area to be treated, with a 3.5- to 5.0-mm spot size set at 1–2 J/cm² most commonly used. Bleeding can occur in these areas as the thermal effect is insufficient to provide hemostasis.

When the erbium laser is the sole utilized system, the first pass is performed to most efficiently debride the epidermis. This is undertaken typically at 100 µm of ablation with no coagulation. The ablation depth is decreased at the periphery to minimize the final demarcation between treated and untreated areas. For the second pass, erbium laser coagulative pulses or, alternatively, ablation with concomitant coagulation is used to provide the heat needed for the tightening effect. Finally, the third pass utilizes the ablation mode to remove superficial necrosis but can also include additional coagulation to enhance the thermal effect. To treat the neck, pure ablation is used with a graduated drop in setting to feather while proceeding lower and laterally on the neck. As with the pulsed CO_2 laser, careful feathering to blend the treated and untreated areas is critical to ensure a natural and cosmetically pleasing result.

Complications of ablative resurfacing can include prolonged erythema, contact dermatitis, acne, infection, pigmentary changes, and scarring (Lewis and Alster 1996; Nanni and Alster 1998; Sriprachya-Anunt 1997). Postoperative erythema typically improves with time; it is most pronounced during the first week and steadily subsides over the next few weeks. Prolonged erythema and/or pruritus result from contact dermatitis, infection, or thermal damage. Allergic and irritant contact dermatitis occurs more commonly in newly resurfaced skin and likely relates to the increased density of Langerhans cells, which is noted in areas of perturbed epidermis. Thus, anything that comes into contact with the skin can trigger a reaction as the disrupted epidermis more readily attracts the dendritic cells to potential sites of antigen invasion. The most likely contactants are sources of perfumes or dyes such as those found in fabric softener dryer sheets or detergents. Patients should be forewarned to eliminate these potential allergens. A reaction to a topical petrolatum-based dressing may occur during the first postoperative week and is best treated by switching to vegetable shortening. Oral antihistamines and topical steroids are invaluable for treating more severe reactions.

Acne can be activated by the occlusive effect of the dressings. It can take up to 6 weeks to clear. This acneform eruption usually responds to removal of the occlusive factor and a topical, or even oral, antibiotic may be needed in more severe cases. After a few weeks, comedolytics such as topical benzoyl peroxide, retinoids, and alpha- or beta-hydroxy acids may be added as needed.

Infection from either a viral, bacterial, or yeast/fungal source can also prolong erythema. Infections need to be treated promptly with a change in oral agents based on culture identification and sensitivity results or based on empiric observation. If herpes simplex viral infection (HSV) is suspected, the antiviral medication should be increased to a herpes zoster dose. Valcyclovir is the antiviral agent of choice, recommended for its ability to attain higher blood levels in comparison to other anti-HSV drugs (Data on file, GlaxoSmithKline). For suspected yeast infections, additional doses of fluconazole or spectazole are recommended.

Relative hypopigmentation can occur when removal of acquired sun damage has returned the skin to its normal nonsun-exposed color. A careful technique of feathering into the untreated, sun-damaged areas will minimize this demarcation. If it is still prominent, a touch up at the line of demarcation can help. Additionally, chemical peeling agents, hydroquinone preparations, or lasers which target melanin can be utilized to minimize the solar lentigines in the untreated area. Delayed hypopigmentation can arise in areas of significant erythema which may mask its earlier appearance. Although this hypopigmentation can be permanent, treatment with the excimer and other similar 308-nm light devices has been shown to improve this leukoderma (Friedman and Geronemus 2001)

Of greatest concern is scarring, which can be atrophic or hypertrophic in nature. Scars should be treated immediately, once they become apparent, as earlier treatment is more beneficial. Topical steroids should be applied and intralesional steroid injection is recommended for any hypertrophic scars. The pulsed dye laser can provide significant benefit but several treatments may be needed to obtain the desired result. The laser settings are similar to those used in other scar treatments and are generally performed at 3- to 6-week intervals, depending on severity, until the scarring process is abated.

Results

Ablative resurfacing leads to dramatic improvement in the overall quality of the skin including fine lines, deeper rhytides, solar lentigos, and elastotic changes. It is also very effective in smoothing other superficial irregularities such as keratoses, nevi, benign tumors, and acne scars (Figs. 5.4–5.6).

The Future

The field of ablative resurfacing has remained stable with relatively few advances over the past 5 years. A notable exception to this has recently arisen with the advent of both plasmakinetic and fractional resurfacing. Although in their infancy, these novel resurfacing techniques show promise as we await the completion of long-term studies.

Nonablative Resurfacing

Currently Available Technology

Currently, the devices which are available in the field of nonablative resurfacing can be divided into two main types: those with a vascular target that initiate a cascade of events by wounding dermal microvasculature and those that target water to deposit heat into the dermis. The first group includes pulsed dye lasers (PDL) and intense pulsed light (IPL) sources, as well as one IPL device used in conjunction with radiofrequency (RF) energy. The pulsed dye lasers are

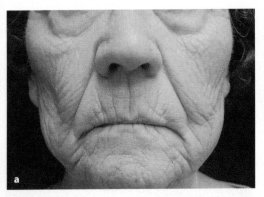
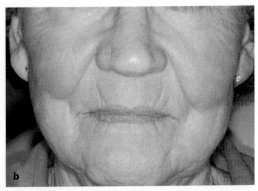

Fig. 5.4. 73-year-old woman with severe dermatoheliosis, pre (a) and 6 weeks post (b) CO_2 and erbium laser resurfacing

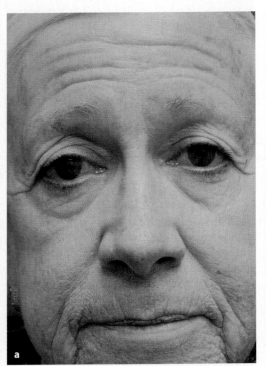
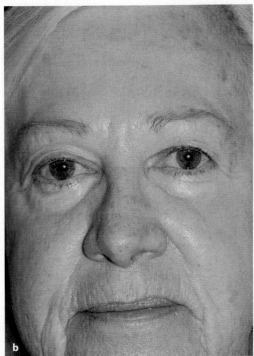

Fig. 5.5. 64-year-old woman with photodamage, pre (a) and post (b) CO_2 laser resurfacing

in the 585- to 595-nm range and have pulse widths which vary from 350–450 ms to 1.5, 3, 6, 10, 20, and 40 ms. IPL sources utilize a broad band of light with cutoff filters in the 550- to 690-nm range which are used to eliminate the shorter, undesirable wavelengths. A recently developed device uses a combination of IPL and RF and has a similar cutoff filter-IPL system with the addition of up to 25 J/cm^3 RF energy. The 1064-nm laser in the millisecond and microsecond domain has been used for nonablative rejuvenation as well. Finally, a combina-

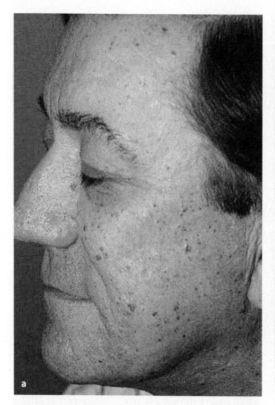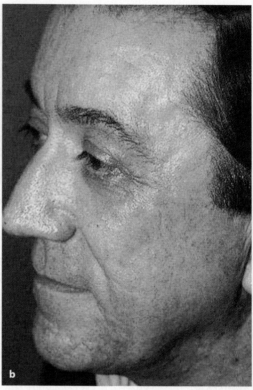

Fig. 5.6. 48-year-old man with dermatosis papulosa nigra, photodamage and acne scarring, pre (**a**) and post (**b**) CO_2 resurfacing

tion treatment with 1064-nm and 532-nm lasers has proven beneficial for fine lines and pigmentary and vascular changes.

There are several mid-infrared lasers that target water to effect dermal heat deposition. The 1320-nm Nd:YAG laser was the original system to use this approach in nonablative resurfacing in conjunction with a spray cooling device to protect the epidermis. Subsequently, the 1450-nm diode laser was shown to have even greater water absorption resulting in more superficial heat deposition. Most recently, the 1540-nm erbium:glass laser system, which has been more widely available in Europe, has emerged as an effective nonablative laser. These devices do not improve vascular or pigmentary changes. However, their histological and clinical improvement of wrinkles is well documented (Fournier et al. 2001; Goldberg et al. 2002; Hardaway 2002; Lupton 2002).

A unique high-powered monopolar RF device has recently been shown to deposit heat deeper in the dermis and possibly into subcutaneous tissue including fascia and fat. This effect can lead to more dramatic tissue tightening as well as traditional nonablative benefits. Additionally, acne scars as well as fine lines and surface changes have been noted to improve (Zelickson 2004).

Advantages

The main advantage of nonablative wrinkle treatment is the relative lack of patient down time in contrast to the obligatory 7–10 days of recovery time for ablative resurfacing. The devices that target dermal vasculature will help minimize, if not eliminate, the telangiectases frequently noted in patients with a history of significant sun exposure. Patients with diffuse erythema, resulting either from sun damage or rosacea, also note improvement. Devices which can target melanin as a potential chromophore, such as those with an IPL component, can also treat any concomitant pigmentary changes. Lentigines, melasma, and poikilodermatous changes can be improved if not completely eradicated.

Disadvantages

The degree of wrinkle reduction is not as significant as that seen with the ablative devices and thus, patient dissatisfaction can be an issue. The improvement is often referred to as skin "toning" or "plumping up of the skin," in contrast to the "tightening" often seen with ablative resurfacing. Appropriate patient education about the degree and unpredictability of enhancement is the key to success for these procedures. Good quality preoperative photography is helpful to document these changes as they can be subtle and improvement occurs over time, making the change less apparent.

Indications

Nonablative resurfacing is best for patients with fine lines, and, if the appropriate device is used, erythema, telangiectasia, or pigmentary changes. Patients with a vascular component are best treated with the longer-pulsed PDLs (VBeam/VStar), IPL, and IPL + RF. IPL is best at targeting pigment and can also target hemoglobin, although multiple treatments are often necessary to eradicate the vascular component. If telangiectases are the more predominant characteristic, the longer-pulsed PDLs are our laser of choice, as they more effectively target vessels in a single treatment and are at least equivalent to IPL devices for wrinkle reduction. For those patients prone to acne or with enlarged pores or sebaceous hyperplasia, the midinfrared systems offer the greatest ability to target the sebaceous gland.

Contraindications

Photosensitivity to the wavelength of light used, recent tan (if using a wavelength absorbed by melanin), and unrealistic expectations are the three main contraindications. In addition, active herpes simplex or other infections or lesions of concern in the treatment field should be avoided.

Consent

Informed consent is mandatory and should include treatment options, potential risks, and benefits. No guarantees should be made. A carefully written, detailed consent that explains the above is suggested (Fig. 5.7).

Personal Laser Technique

The wide array of nonablative rejuvenation devices allows us to individualize treatment based on patients' specific concerns. If vessels and pigment are the main issues, we start by targeting the chromophore most bothersome to the patient. Subsequently, we use the system which would best treat the most prominent residual chromophore. For the pulsed dye lasers, using the largest spot size with the highest fluence at a pulse width that is just subpurpuric provides the best results. Typical PDL settings include a 10-mm spot size with 7–7.5 J/cm^2 and a 6-ms pulse width. Occasionally, we will increase the pulse width to 10 ms to avoid purpura if the patient is on some form of anticoagulant therapy. One pass is performed for nonablative rejuvenation, whereas additional pulses may be needed to treat discrete vessels, if present.

For mild, diffuse erythema, especially when lentigines are also present, we start with an IPL device, as it will target both melanin and hemoglobin. IPL sources vary depending on the flash lamp and the cut-off filters used. The spot size is usually set, but the pulse width can be varied by time per pulse and spacing between 1 and 3 pulses.

Although a 585-nm, 350-ms PDL is used for wrinkle reduction, the low utilized fluences of

Consent for Nonablative Resurfacing/Collagen Stimulation

These lasers use a light to selectively heat up the collagen in the dermis to stimulate collagen remodeling. The superficial part of the skin is spared; therefore, there is no injury to the outer layers of skin. This means that there will be no break in the *surface* of the skin and you can apply makeup immediately after laser treatment. There is little or no downtime associated with this laser treatment. Because there is no improvement in the superficial part of the skin, patients often do microdermabrasion in conjunction with laser treatment to help smooth out some of the fine lines and pigmentary changes that can be seen. Microdermabrasion also helps by removing outer most layers of skin, which allows better penetration of any topical treatment that you are using.

Other alternatives include microdermabrasion alone, chemical peels or laser resurfacing. Ablative laser resurfacing differs from nonablative resurfacing in that it physically removes the outer portions of the skin, and usually causes immediate tightening of the skin. With laser resurfacing you have more improvement in the outer layers with removal of sun damage changes and more tightening, but an additional 1 week period of down time. Both ablative and nonablative techniques lead to new collagen formation which continues for at least 6 months. Microdermabrasion alone will improve some of the fine lines on the surface of the skin and some of the pigmentary changes, but will not produce significant collagen remodeling or skin tightening.

Although rare, potential complications of laser treatment include pigmentary changes or scarring. As with any injury to the skin, there is a potential for poor healing.

Typically 2–5 treatments are performed at one month intervals and the resulting increase in collagen formation will continue for six months so that maximum benefits may not be noted for six to eight months after this procedure.

NO GUARANTEES

It is possible that you may derive no benefits from the above described procedure. While this procedure is effective in most cases, no guarantees can be made that a specific patient will benefit from treatment. Do not sign this form unless you have had a chance to ask questions and have received satisfactory answers to all of your questions.

WAIVER OF LIABILITY

All insurance companies, including Medicare, only pay for services that they determine to be 'reasonable' and necessary. If your insurance company determines that a particular service is not reasonable and necessary under their program standards, they will deny payment for that service. **I believe that your insurance, or Medicare, will deny payment for the following reason: Insurances usually do not pay for cosmetic procedures.**

CONSENT

MY SIGNATURE INDICATES THE FOLLOWING: 1) I HAVE READ AND I UNDERSTAND THE INFORMATION OUTLINED ABOVE; 2) I HAVE DISCUSSED MY QUESTIONS WITH THE DOCTOR OR HER STAFF.

I AUTHORIZE THE RELEASE OF MY PHOTOGRAPHS.

DATE . . . . NAME OF PATIENT . . . . SIGNATURE OF PATIENT . . . .

DATE . . . . NAME OF STAFF . . . . SIGNATURE OF STAFF . . . .

Fig. 5.7. Informed consent for nonablative resurfacing

3 J/cm² with a 7-mm spot size does not effectively target vasculature. When the laser is used with a 5-mm spot size and higher fluences, vasculature can also be treated.

The most commonly used 1320-nm Nd:YAG laser is used with a spray cooling device that provides not only pre-, but also mid- and postcooling of the epidermis to allow for a more superficial level of skin treatment. A temperature sensor reads the surface heat generated by a test pulse and the goal is to keep it in the 40°C to 45°C range. Energy settings are then set accordingly. Although originally done with a single pass, three passes are now recommended utilizing a precooling pass, a midcooling pass, and a postcooling pass. The precooling pass is performed at 30 ms cooling duration with a fluence range of 14–18 J/cm², which is based on temperature sensor readings. The midcooling pass is used in combination with pre- and postcooling at the following settings: 5-ms precool, 5-ms midcool, and 20-ms postcool at 17 J/cm². The postcooling pass fluences are adjusted based on temperature sensor readings and range from 13 to 17 J/cm² with a 30-ms postcool duration.

The 1450-nm midinfrared laser has greater water absorption so changes noted are more superficial. This may be more advantageous in targeting dermal solar damage, which typically involves the superficial dermis. It is used with a similar dynamic cooling device that protects the epidermis while depositing the heat in the dermis. When used for nonablative rejuvenation, the larger 6-mm hand piece is used typically at 10–16 J/cm² with cooling at 25–35 ms. To target a specific lesion, as in sebaceous hyperplasia, the 4-mm spot is used and the fluence is increased to 17–18 J/cm² and cooling is decreased to 30 ms. Larger lesions can even be double pulsed.

Postoperative Care and Complications

Minimal postoperative care is needed as the epidermis remains intact. Mild burning, erythema, and edema can occur, and the application of aloe vera gel and/or ice packs is helpful. Bruising may occur when pulsed dye lasers are used at the shorter pulse widths; this can usually be covered with makeup.

Complications are unusual and much less likely than with ablative techniques where epidermal disruption leaves an entryway for bacteria and other contactants. Tanned skin will be more susceptible to injury due to the increased melanin absorption if wavelengths absorbed by melanin are used and the epidermis is insufficiently cooled. Use of too high an energy setting can lead to hyperpigmentation or burning and blistering. Hypopigmentation, and even scarring, has been reported (Gaston and Clark 1998; Hardaway 2002; Menaker 1999; Moreno-Arias 2002; Wlotzke 1996).

Results

Results vary among individuals. Nearly all patients who have undergone biopsies after nonablative resurfacing have shown histological improvement with increased number of fibroblasts, increased collagen deposition, and normalization of the papillary dermis (Fitzpatrick et al. 2000; Goldberg 1999). Clinical improvement, however, can be more subtle and does not appear to correlate with histological improvement. Although results are relatively inconspicuous and occur slowly over time, most patients concur that the skin feels "tighter," "firmer," and more "toned" (Figs. 5.8–5.11).

The Future

The field of nonablative resurfacing has expanded dramatically over the past 8 years. Studies are underway to elucidate the best treatment intervals, compare the above techniques, and expand the energy potential of the given devices. In addition, a new 900-nm laser in conjunction with RF shows promise.

5

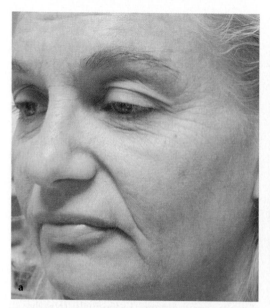 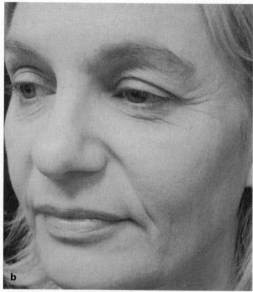

Fig. 5.8. 50-year-old woman with deepened nasolabial groove, pre (**a**) and 4 months post (**b**) a single full-face unipolar radiofrequency nonablative treatment

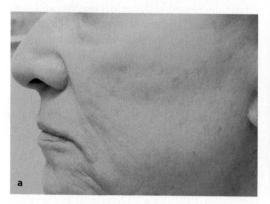 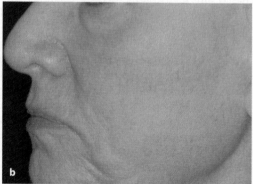

Fig. 5.9. 69-year-old woman with acne scarring, telangiectases, and wrinkles, pre (**a**) and 4 months post (**b**) PDL treatment

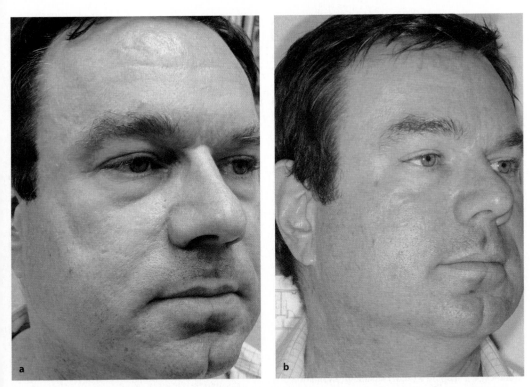

Fig. 5.10. 44-year-old man with acne scarring and sebaceous hyperplasia, pre (**a**) and 4 months post (**b**) 1450-nm diode laser treatment

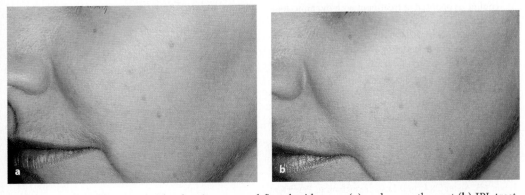

Fig. 5.11. 36-year-old woman with telangiectases and fine rhytides, pre (**a**) and 4 months post (**b**) IPL treatment

5

References

Christian MM, Behroozan DS, Moy RL (2000) Delayed infections following full-face CO_2 laser resurfacing and occlusive dressing use. Dermatol Surg 26(1):32–36

Fitzpatrick RE, Rostan EF, Marchell N (2000) Collagen tightening induced by carbon dioxide laser versus erbium: YAG laser. Lasers Surg Med 27(5):395–403

Fournier N, Dahan S, Barneon G, Diridollou S, Lagarde JM, Gall Y, Mordon S (2001) Nonablative remodeling: clinical, histologic, ultrasound imaging, and profilometric evaluation of a 1540-nm Er:glass laser. Dermatol Surg 27(9):799–806

Friedman PM, Geronemus RG (2001) Use of the 308-nm excimer laser for postresurfacing leukoderma. Arch Dermatol 137(6):824–825

Gaston DA, Clark DP (1998) Facial hypertrophic scarring from pulsed dye laser. Dermatol Surg 24(5): 523–525

Goldberg DJ (1999) Non-ablative subsurface remodeling: clinical and histologic evaluation of a 1320-nm Nd:YAG laser. J Cutan Laser Ther 1(3):153–157

Goldberg DJ (2000) New collagen formation after dermal remodeling with an intense pulsed light source. J Cutan Laser Ther 2(2):59–61

Goldberg DJ, Silapunt S (2001) Histologic evaluation of a Q-switched Nd:YAG laser in the nonablative treatment of wrinkles. Dermatol Surg 27(8):744–746

Goldberg DJ, Rogachefsky AS, Silapunt S (2002) Nonablative laser treatment of facial rhytides: a comparison of 1450-nm diode laser treatment with dynamic cooling as opposed to treatment with dynamic cooling alone. Lasers Surg Med 30(2):79–81

Hardaway CA, Ross EV, Paithankar DY (2002) Non-ablative cutaneous remodeling with a 1.45 microM mid-infrared diode laser: phase II. J Cosmet Laser Ther 4(1):9–14

Kilmer SL, Chotzen V, Zelickson BD, McClaren M, Silva S, Calkin J, No D (2003) Full-face laser resurfacing using a supplemented topical anesthesia protocol. Arch Dermatol 139(10):1279–1283

Lask G, Keller G, Lowe N, Gormley D (1995) Laser skin resurfacing with the SilkTouch flashscanner for facial rhytides. Dermatol Surg 21(12):1021–1024

Lewis AB, Alster TS (1996) Laser resurfacing: Persistent erythema and postinflammatory hyperpigmentation. J Geriatr Dermatol 4:75–76

Lupton JR, Williams CM, Alster TS (2002) Nonablative laser skin resurfacing using a 1540-nm erbium glass laser: a clinical and histologic analysis. Dermatol Surg 28(9):833–835

Menaker GM, Wrone DA, Williams RM, Moy RL (1999) Treatment of facial rhytides with a nonablative laser: a clinical and histologic study. Dermatol Surg 25(6):440–444

Nanni CA, Alster TS (1998) Complications of carbon dioxide laser resurfacing: An evaluation of 500 patients. Dermatol Surg 24:209–219

Pozner JM, Goldberg DJ (2000) Histologic effect of a variable pulsed Er:YAG laser. Dermatol Surg 26(8): 733–736

Sriprachya-Anunt S, Goldman MP, Fitzpatrick RE, Goldman MP, et al. (1997) Infections complicating pulsed carbon dioxide laser resurfacing for photoaged facial skin. Dermatol Surg 23:527–536

Sriprachya-Anunt S, Marchell NL, Fitzpatrick RE, Goldman MP, Rostan EF (2002) Facial resurfacing in patients with Fitzpatrick skin type IV. Lasers Surg Med 30(2):86–92

Tanzi EL, Alster TS (2003) Side effects and complications of variable-pulsed erbium:yttrium-aluminum-garnet laser skin resurfacing: extended experience with 50 patients. Plast Reconstr Surg 111(4):1524–1529; discussion 1530–1532

Wlotzke U, Hohenleutner U, Abd-El-Raheem TA, Baumler W, Landthaler M (1996) Side-effects and complications of flashlamp-pumped pulsed dye laser therapy of port-wine stains. A prospective study. Br J Dermatol 134(3):475–480

Zachary CB (2000) Modulating the Er:YAG laser. Lasers Surg Med 26(2):223–226

Zelickson BD, Kilmer SL, Bernstein E, Chotzen VA, Dock J, Mehregan D, Coles C (1999) Pulsed dye laser therapy for sun damaged skin. Lasers Surg Med 25(3):229–236

Zelickson BD, Kist D, Bernstein E, Brown DB, Ksenzenko S, Burns J, Kilmer S, Mehregan D, Pope K (2004) Histological and ultrastructural evaluation of the effects of a radiofrequency-based nonablative dermal remodeling device: a pilot study. Arch Dermatol 140(2):204–209

Lasers, Photodynamic Therapy, and the Treatment of Medical Dermatologic Conditions

Michael H. Gold

Core Messages

- Lasers and light sources have become more commonplace in the treatment of dermatologic medical diseases.
- ALA-PDT is a proven therapy for actinic keratoses and superficial nonmelanoma skin cancers.
- ALA-PDT is being used to treat the signs of photorejuvenation with a variety of vascular lasers, blue light sources, and the intense pulsed light source.
- ALA-PDT, with blue light, is a useful therapy for acne vulgaris.
- ALA-PDT is being used to treat moderate to severe acne vulgaris, and other sebaceous gland disorders with a variety of vascular lasers, blue light sources, and the intense pulsed light source.
- New lasers and light sources are being used to treat psoriasis vulgaris, vitiligo, other disorders of pigmentation, and hypopigmented stretch marks.

History of Photodynamic Therapy

The treatment of superficial nonmelanoma skin cancers and actinic keratoses (AKs) with lasers and light sources has recently entered a new era in dermatology with the advent of 20% 5-aminolevulinic acid (ALA), a potent photosensitizer. This photosensitizer has demonstrated an effective ability to interact with lasers and light sources of appropriate wavelengths to selectively destroy the lesions in question. The

term photodynamic therapy, or PDT, is now a phrase which is not foreign to laser physicians and has, over the past several years, become an integral part of their therapeutic armamentarium. A review of what PDT is, its history and how it is being incorporated into dermatologist's offices today will follow.

PDT is a treatment modality which involves the use of a photosensitizer, a light source which fits the absorption spectrum of the photosensitizer, and molecular oxygen, which when stimulated will destroy a specific target tissue. To be effective in the process, the photosensitizer must be able to preferentially penetrate more into the targeted tissue than the surrounding skin. ALA has been shown to be absorbed very well by actinically damaged skin, skin cancer cells, and by the pilosebaceous glands of the skin. The photosensitizer may be given exogenously or formed endogenously during normal biochemical pathways found within certain disease state pathways. An appropriate light source must be employed to activate the photosensitizer and the wavelength of that light must be within the appropriate absorption spectrum of the photosensitizer. Various lasers and light are being utilized by dermatologists for PDT. These devices have different wavelengths of light and thus different penetration depths into tissues.

5-ALA, the most common drug used in dermatology for PDT, occurs naturally in cells as an intermediate product formed during the endogenous porphyrin synthesis process. 5-ALA acts as a "prodrug" and has been demonstrated to effectively penetrate the stratum corneum and to localize in the target tissues already mentioned. Once localized into the appropriate cells within the target tissues, the 5-ALA is transformed into a highly photoactive

Fig. 6.1.

Protoporphyrin absorption
spectrum

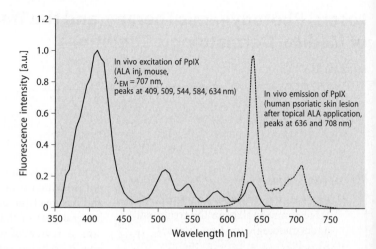

6

endogenous porphyrin derivative, protoporphyrin IX (PpIX), which has an absorption spectrum of light in the 415- to 630-nm range (Fig. 6.1).

The history of PDT can trace its routes back to 1900 when Raab (Kalka 2000) found that Paramecium caudatum cells died quickly when exposed to light in the presence of acridine orange. In 1904, this process was first described as the "photodynamic effect." This work involved the study of protozoa and described oxygen-consuming chemical reactions and fluorescence patterns after the applications of analine dyes. In 1905 5% eosin was first utilized as a skin photosensitizer. Artificial light was used to successfully treat human nonmelanoma skin cancer, condylomata lata, and lupus vulgaris. The next forty-odd years found very few substantial studies being described using PDT.

In 1948, hematoporphyrin was found to be selectively absorbed in neoplastic tissues, embryonic tissues, and traumatized tissues. This work led to the development of a purified synthetic compound, a hematoporphyrin derivative, which then became the standard for PDT research and treatment in that time. Dougherty et al. (Dougherty et al. 1978) reported in 1978 the use of this hematoporphyrin derivative and its photoactivation with a red light source. This group described its effectiveness in treating a variety of cutaneous malignancies and other cancers as well. PDT has been studied and continues to be investigated for its role in treating a

variety of malignancies including lung, colon, esophagus, peritoneum, pleura, gastrointestinal tract, brain, eye, and skin (Rowe 1988). A variety of nononcologic applications utilizing PDT includes atherosclerosis, infectious diseases, and rheumatologic diseases, as well as skin concerns where the pilosebaceous units are involved. Svaasand (Svassand et al. 1996) described a dosimetry model for PDT which further delineated the necessary three steps for the PDT process to occur: (1) ALA diffusion through the stratum corneum and ability to penetrate the epidermis and dermis, (2) synthesis and production of the photosensitive PpIX from the exogenous ALA applied to the skin, and (3) the production of singlet oxygen when PpIX is properly irradiated with a wavelength of light which is absorbed by PpIX.

In the United States, PDT therapy emerged in the late 1990s as a treatment for nonhyperkeratotic AKs of the face and scalp. AKs are a problem which dermatologists encounter on a daily basis in their clinical practices. The Actinic Keratosis Consensus Conference of 2001 reported that AKs serve as a marker for photodamage and that their principle etiology is ultraviolet light, specifically ultraviolet B light. They found that AKs are associated with alterations of DNA that are associated with squamous cell carcinomas (SCCs), specifically mutations in the tumor-suppressing gene *p53*.

The conference reported that AKs are a carcinoma in situ and some of them will naturally

Table 6.1. Treatment options for actinic keratoses

Surgical options for AK treatment
  Cryosurgery
  Curettage
  Excisional surgery
  Diffuse superficial destructive processes
    Chemical peels
    Dermabrasion
    Laser resurfacing
  ALA-PDT photodynamic therapy
Medical treatments for AKs
  5-Fluorouracil
  Imiquimod
  Retinoids – tretinoin, adapalene, tazarotene
  Dicofenac

regress, some will remain stable, or some will progress to the formation of SCCs. Which will regress or which will progress cannot as yet be determined. The natural history of AKs is unpredictable, and therefore all AKs should be treated in some fashion to prevent the potential onset of cutaneous malignancies. Conversion rates to SCCs have been reported from 0.1% to 20%. Additionally, 97% of SCCs are associated with a nearby AK. Nearby AKs have been found in 44% of cutaneous SCCs which had metastasized. These findings also support the concept that all AKs should be treated to prevent further potential conversion to SCCs.

A variety of treatment options are currently available for the treatment of AKs. These include both medical and surgical options (Table 6.1). Most contend that the principle treatment for AKs involve a destructive process. ALA-PDT fits nicely into this destructive category for the treatment of AKs and has received a great deal of recent attention for its role in the treatment of AKs and other cutaneous concerns.

In Europe, ALA research has focused on its use in treating not only AKs but also for the treatment of superficial cutaneous malignancies. These malignancies include squamous cell carcinoma in situ (Bowen's Disease) basal (BCCs) and squamous cell carcinomas. Numerous clinical reports have now described this role for PDT (Lui and Anderson 1993). A variety of lasers and light sources have been used to treat AKs, Bowen's Dis-

ease, BCCs, and SCCs. For AKs, response rates from 80% to 100% are routinely reported. For Bowen's Disease, response rates from 90% to 100% are reported with PDT. For BCCs and SCCs, 67%–100% of treated lesions respond to PDT. A variety of treatment protocols have been utilized but most have used multiple treatment applications with sufficient follow-up to document the effectiveness of ALA-PDT in the treatment of cutaneous malignancies.

Currently Available Technology

The two main photosensitizers being utilized in this time frame are 20% 5-ALA, known as Levulan, manufactured by Dusa Pharmaceuticals, Wilmington, MA, and the methyl-ester derivative of 5-ALA, Metvix, made by PhotoCure ASA, Norway. Both of these compounds have received extensive study over the last several years and will be summarized below.

Photodynamic Therapy: The Experience with Actinic Keratoses in the United States

In the United States, the 20% 5-ALA product is currently the only commercial product available for use by physicians. It is a 20% weight/volume ALA solution with 48% ethanol. It is produced in the form of a kerastick (Fig. 6.2). The kerastick has a dermatologic applicator at one of its ends for accurate application of the ALA medicine. The applicator tip is attached to flexible plastic tubing which contains two glass vials. One of the vials contains the ALA in a powder form and the other glass vial contains the ethanol solvent. The vials on the kerastick are broken by light manual pressure to the tubing and then the contents are mixed by rotating the contents of the kerastick back and forth for several minutes, with 3 min being the recommended time frame for proper mixing of the medicine. Once fully mixed together, the ALA is ready for patient application. Preparation of the patient includes washing of the skin with a mild cleanser followed by one or two applications of the ALA. Some clinicians advocate the use of an acetone scrub or a microdermabrasion procedure to allow an even deeper penetration of the ALA. Once the drug has been incubated for the time period chosen, the ALA is washed off the skin and the patient is then ready for the appropriate light therapy.

The first clinical trial with 20% 5-ALA was a Phase II clinical trial reported in 2001. In this clinical trial, 36 individuals with nonhyperkeratotic AKs of the face and scalp were evaluated for its safety and efficacy. The patients had the ALA applied to individual AK lesions. The drug was allowed to incubate on the individual lesions for 14–18 h without occlusion and the patient was then subjected to a blue light source

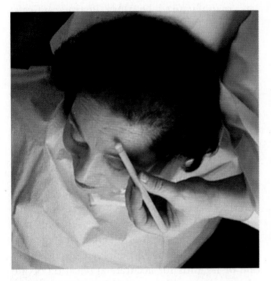

Fig. 6.2. 20% topical ALA

(wavelengths of 410–430 nm) for 16 min and 40 sec. The blue light source provided a dose of 10 J/cm² to the affected lesions. The results of the trial showed that nonhyperkeratotic AKs were effectively treated with the ALA-PDT plus the blue light source. Specifically, 66% of the treated AKs responded to the therapy after one treatment. For those AKs which did not respond ($n=16$), retreatment was undertaken after 8 weeks. This improved the efficacy rate to 85% at the 16-week follow-up period. The treatments were well tolerated by the participants in this trial. All patients noted burning and stinging during their light therapy, and facial erythema was reported in 96% of the participants; all resolved by the first 4-week follow-up.

This aforementioned study led to the Phase III clinical trial, which was a placebo-controlled multicenter analysis looking at a larger number of individuals ($n=243$) using a similar protocol as reported in the Phase II trial. Two applications of either the ALA solution (L) or a vehicle placebo (V) were applied to the individual AK lesions, incubation times for the drug remained at 14–18 h, and the patients received 16 min, 40 s of blue light therapy. Results of the clinical trials showed significant differences between the active ALA and the placebo (Fig. 6.3); more than 70% of the lesions were resolved at 12 weeks. Lesions which were not clear were retreated at 8 weeks. At the conclusion of the study, 88% of the patients with active medicine had a ≥75% response rate compared to 20% in the vehicle/ placebo group of patients. (Fig. 6.4). The treatments were well tolerated by the study partici-

Fig. 6.3.
Levulan PDT system
Phase III studies: efficacy
results. $p < 0.001$.
From Dusa Pharmaceuticals

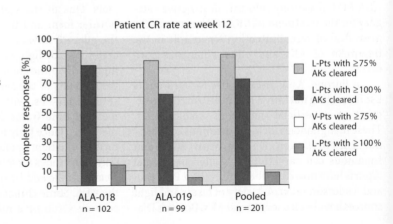

Patient CR rate at week 12

Legend:
- L-Pts with ≥75% AKs cleared
- L-Pts with ≥100% AKs cleared
- V-Pts with ≥75% AKs cleared
- L-Pts with ≥100% AKs cleared

pants. Patients noted that during their light therapy, there was stinging and burning. Some of the patients did have associated erythema and edema from the therapy. These symptoms resolved at 1 week after the light treatment. No noncutaneous adverse effects were seen in the Phase III trials. An important outcome of this trial was patient and physician assessment of improvement in the cosmetic appearance of the skin as a result of the ALA therapies. Ninety four percent of the patients and 92% of the investigators rated the cosmetic improvement as good to excellent.

Recently, a long-term clinical trial has looked at both efficacy and recurrence rates associated with ALA therapy. This study showed that 69% of 32 AKs studied in four individuals remained clear at the end of 4 years; 9% were found to be recurrent; 22% were described as "uncertain" as to whether the lesions were actually recurrent or whether new lesions developed in the same area.

Photodynamic Therapy: New Indications for Photodynamic Photorejuvenation in the United States

We have also studied the use of 20% 5-ALA for AKs with the blue light source. This study looked at the role of ALA-PDT for photoaging (Figs. 6.5, 6.6). Recently, others have begun to explore new ways to revise our current mind-

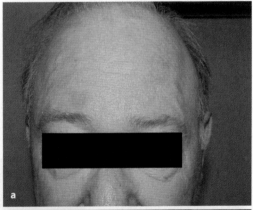

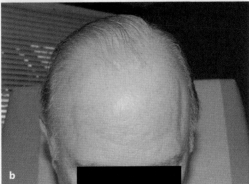

Fig. 6.4. **a** Pretreatment. **b** One week after ALA-PDT treatment. **c** One month after ALA-PDT treatment

Fig. 6.5. **a** Immediately after blue light treatment. **b** One month after treatment

set on the proper use of this therapy for photoaging and photorejuvenation. Such studies have included the use of broad application of the ALA over the entire area which will be treated, and the use of a variety of lasers and light sources which fit the absorption spectrum of protoporphyrin IX (Fig. 6.1). The light sources which are being studied include a variety of blue light sources, the pulsed dye vascular lasers, and myriad different intense pulsed light (IPL) devices (Table 6.2). In addition, shorter drug incubation times, with the average being 1 h, are now routinely being employed to help make the procedures more accessible to the patients being treated. This means that the patients need only to have therapy on one day versus two consecutive days. In addition, with newer light sources, therapy becomes more tolerable to the patients by potentially lessening the adverse effect profile seen with the original Phase II and Phase III trial patients.

To support the notion of full-face, short-contact ALA therapy, a number of clinical investigators have recently reported their successes with ALA for photorejuvenation. Photorejuvenation utilizing lasers and light sources has been successfully utilized over the past several years to noninvasively rejuvenate the skin, improving facial telangiectasias, pigmentary dyschromias, and overall skin texture. Ruiz-Rodriquez et al. (Ruiz-Rodriquez et al. 2002) found that after 4 h of drug incubation, patients responded well to

Table 6.2. Lasers/light sources currently being used for photorejuvenation with 20% 5-ALA

Blue light sources
  Blue U (Dusa Pharmaceuticals)
  ClearLight (CureLight, Lumenis)
Pulsed dye vascular lasers
  V-Star (Cynosure)
  V-Beam (Candela)
Intense pulsed light sources
  Quantum, Vasculight (Lumenis)
  Aurora (Syneron)
  ClearTouch, SkinStation (Radiancy)
  Estelux, Medilux (Palomar)

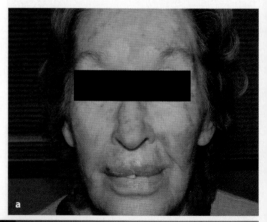

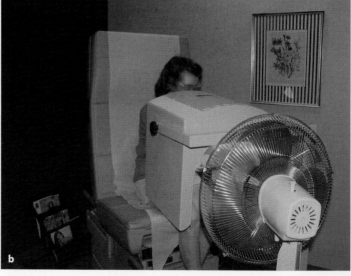

Fig. 6.6.
a Before ALA-PDT blue light therapy. **b** Patient undergoing 4th ALA-PDT blue light therapy session

ALA therapy. In addition, skin quality improvement and a decrease in AKs were noted. Seventeen individuals were studied in this trial with 38 AKs being assessed. Two IPL sessions with ALA applied for 4 h yielded excellent cosmetic results and an 87% improvement in the parameters of photorejuvenation (wrinkling, skin texture, pigmentary changes, and telangiectasias). He called this new therapeutic approach "photodynamic photorejuvenation," a term which fully describes the use of ALA-PDT and lasers and light sources. Another study utilized IPL therapy with ALA in 18 individuals with full-face, short-contact therapy. In this study incubation of the ALA was undertaken for 1, 2, and 3 h followed by exposure to a blue light source. The investigators found that 1-h drug incubation was as efficacious as the original 14- to 18-h drug incubation time periods. The patients showed improvement in skin sallowness, fine wrinkling, and mottled hyperpigmentation with this therapy. Gold (Gold 2003) reported his experience with full-face, short-contact ALA therapy with IPL in ten patients. IPL settings included the use of a 550-nm cut-off filter, double pulsing with a 3.5-ms pulse delay, and fluence ranges from 20 to 34 J/cm². The patients in this clinical trial received 3 monthly IPL treatments and had follow-up visits at 1 and 3 months following the last IPL therapy. Results from this clinical trial showed that over 85% of the targeted AKs responded to the therapy. In addition, there was a global skin quality improvement score of greater than 75% compared to the baseline visits.

Furthermore, there was a 90% improvement in crow's feet, 100% improvement in tactile skin roughness, 90% improvement in mottled hyperpigmentation, and a 70% improvement in facial erythema. No adverse effects were reported; 30% did have facial erythema and edema reported immediately after therapy which abated within 24–48 h. No patient in this clinical investigation reported any downtime from their day-to-day activities as a result of their therapies. (Figs. 6.7, 6.8). Other investigators (Goldman et al. 2002) evaluated 32 patients with moderate photodamage and multiple AKs, again using full-face, short-contact therapy and the blue light source. At the end of this clinical trial there was a 90% clearance of AKs, a 72% improvement in skin texture, and a 59% improvement in skin pigmentation. Of note, 62.5% of the patients in this trial found this therapy less painful than cryotherapy. Avram and Goldman (Avram and Goldman 2004) reported on 17 individuals using full-face, short-contact ALA therapy and one IPL treatment. They used 1-h drug incubation and found that 68% of the AKs treated responded after the one IPL treatment. In addition, they found that there was a 55% improvement in facial telangiectasias, 48% improvement in pigmentary irregularities, and 25% improvement in skin texture, all with just one PDT treatment.

The pulse dye laser has also been shown to be useful in the photorejuvenation of the skin. By utilizing ALA, Alexiades-Armenakas et al. (Alexiades-Armenakas and Geronemus 2003), evaluated both 3-h and 14- to 18-h drug incuba-

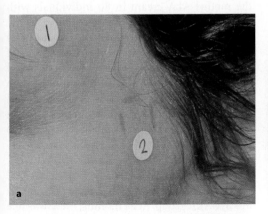 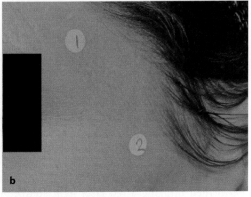

Fig. 6.7. a AK before ALA-PDT/IPL therapy. b AK area 1 month after ALA-PDT/IPL therapy

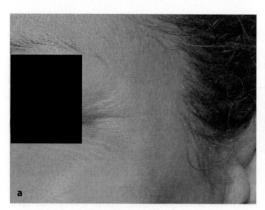
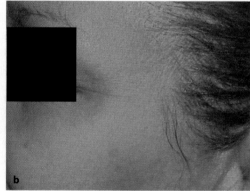

Fig. 6.8. **a** Crows feet immediately after ALA-PDT/IPL therapy. **b** Crows feet 1 month after ALA-PDT/IPL therapy

tions. They found both incubation periods successful in treating AKs and in improving the parameters of photorejuvenation. This group utilized a pulsed dye laser at 595 nm, with fluence ranges of 4–7.5 J/cm², 10-ms pulse durations, 10-mm spot size and 30-ms cryogen sprays. They evaluated 2,561 face and scalp AKs with clearances of 99.9% at 10 days, 94.8% at 2 months, and 90.1% at 4 months. Trunk lesions were also evaluated; 54.5% responded at 10 days and 74.4% at 2 months.

Finally, another study has looked at the safety and efficacy of large-surface application of ALA in hairless mice. In this study investigators looked at blue light therapy alone, ALA therapy alone, and the combination of ALA and blue light with weekly applications being performed for 10 months. No tumors were formed during this trial period; therefore ALA-PDT should be deemed not only efficacious but safe as well.

Photodynamic Therapy: The (Primarily) European Experience with Actinic Keratoses and Skin Cancers

The methyl ester derivative of ALA, known as Metvix, is available in Europe and several other countries, and is currently undergoing clinical evaluations in the United States. Many trials evaluating the methyl ester of ALA have been performed utilizing a red laser light source at 630 nm (Fig. 6.1). This approach led to European Union approval for the treatment of non-hyperkeratotic AKs of the face and scalp as well as BCCs which are unsuitable for conventional therapy. Recommendations for the use of the methyl-ALA include the gentle scraping or curettage of the effected lesion prior to the application of the methyl-ALA cream. This is then occluded for 3 h before the cream is removed and the area is subjected to the red laser light source. Several recent clinical trials support the use of the methyl-ALA in the treatment of AKs. In one study, investigators studied 204 individuals treated with the methyl-ALA cream as compared to cryotherapy and placebo. The methyl-ALA technique was found to have better response rates and cosmetic improvement compared to both cryotherapy and placebo. In another study, investigators studied the methyl-ALA cream in 80 individuals with AKs. They found an 89% improvement in the AKs and a 90% improvement in the cosmetic appearance. In their group of patients, 72% of them preferred PDT over both cryotherapy and 5-FU therapy. Others recently completed a prospective randomized study of BCCs treated with either methyl-ALA or surgery in 101 patients. After 3 months of follow-up, there was a 98% complete response rate with surgery versus a 91% response rate with the methyl-ALA. After 12 months, there was a 96% response rate with surgery and an 83% response seen in the methyl-ALA group. At 24 months, there was one recurrence noted in the surgery group and 5 in the methyl-ALA group. The authors concluded that the cosmetic appearance was better in the methyl-ALA group compared to the surgical group.

ALA-PDT is a new therapeutic modality to enhance previously accepted lasers and light source technologies. With short-contact, topical ALA full-face treatments, it appears that all parameters of photorejuvenation and associated AKs can be successfully treated with a reduced number of treatments. The exact number of required therapeutic sessions has yet to be determined. Most clinicians perform one to three sessions at 1-month intervals. Adverse events are kept to a minimum. Patients routinely report no downtime from day-to-day activities utilizing ALA-PDT in this manner. Further research is required to further validate and define this new therapy for photorejuvenation and associated AKs.

Photodynamic Therapy – Other Indications

The use of ALA-PDT is not limited to the treatment of AKs, BCCs, and SCCs. PDT therapy has long been recognized as an important treatment in acne vulgaris and other disorders of the pilosebaceous glands. Recent advances have made the use of a variety of lasers and light sources combined with ALA practical for those suffering from acne vulgaris and other pilosebaceous entities.

■ Acne Vulgaris

Acne vulgaris accounts for over 30% of all dermatology visits. It has been estimated that between 70% and 96% of all individuals will suffer from acne vulgaris at some point in their lifetime. Recent evidence suggests that over 40 million American adolescents and 25 million American adults are affected by acne vulgaris.

In its simplest form, acne vulgaris is a disorder of the sebaceous glands. Obstruction of the sebaceous glands leads to the production and proliferation of bacterial growth within the sebaceous glands. The bacteria most commonly associated with the formation of acne vulgaris is *Propionobacterium acnes (P. acnes)*. Inflammatory acne presents with papules, pustules, and cysts.

There are a variety of effective medications to treat those individuals suffering from acne vulgaris. These include topical and systemic antibiotics, topical benzoyl peroxide, topical salicylic acid derivatives, and a variety of topical sulfa preparations. Topical and systemic retinoids round out the successful medications for the treatment of acne vulgaris. Despite continuing advances, there are drawbacks to each group of therapies. Some of the topical medications are irritating to the skin and may cause clothes to stain. Most topical therapies are slow to achieve an acceptable onset of action, some requiring several months to become successful. Systemic antibiotics, the mainstay for inflammatory acne for many years, have recently been reported to show up to a 40% drug resistance with the commonly used oral tetracyclines, erythromycins, and sulfa derivatives. A recent report has even suggested that the long-term use of systemic antibiotics in women may be associated with a higher incidence of breast cancer (Velicer et al. 2004).

Exposure to natural and artificial UV light has been reported to be successful in the treatment of acne vulgaris (Sigurdsson et al. 1997). The exact mechanism for this response of acneform lesions to UV light is not fully understood but is felt to be due, in part, to destruction of *P. acnes* bacteria in the sebaceous unit. This natural endogenous PDT reaction works well in the treatment of acne vulgaris; however, the damaging effects of UV light with regard to photoaging and the development of skin cancers precludes its regular use in today's medical environment.

The photodynamic reaction seen in the destruction of the *P. acnes* bacteria involves the natural production of porphyrins seen during the growth of the *P. acnes* during the inflammatory phase of the acne cycle. The porphyrins produced are principally PpIX and Coproporphyrin III, which have absorption spectra in the near ultraviolet range of light, in the blue light range, with peak absorption seen at 415 nm. The PDT reaction leads to photoactivation of the *P. acnes'* porphyrins after exposure to the appropriate light source. This causes the formation of singlet oxygen within the bacteria. Ultimately, destruction of the *P. acnes* bacteria will occur, with resultant destruction of the acne lesion, leaving surrounding tissues and structures fully intact.

A variety of light sources have been used over the past century to treat acne vulgaris. These have included halogen, xenon, and tungsten light sources. More recently, investigations have focused predominantly on blue light and ALA, blue light alone, vascular lasers, and a variety of light sources. These lasers and light sources all utilize the concept of PDT and the destruction of the *P. acnes*. Still other lasers focus on destruction of the sebaceous gland and sebaceous gland activity output. Both groups will be reviewed.

The treatment of inflammatory acne vulgaris with blue light sources has been extensively reviewed over the past several years. Papageorgiou (Papageorgiou et al. 2000) reported his findings with a blue light source. He showed that 63% of inflammatory lesions responded to blue light and 45% of comedonal lesions also responded. Other investigators showed that 65% of inflammatory acne lesions responded to blue light therapy. A new high-intensity blue light source has also recently been evaluated for its effectiveness in the treatment of inflammatory acne vulgaris (Elman et al. 2003). Investigators have shown between 60% and 75% improvement with this high-intensity blue light source. Most of the clinical trials have evaluated two treatments per week for 4 weeks with appropriate 1- and 3-month follow-ups. These clinical trials had, on average, a 20% nonresponder rate. Gold (Gold 2003) reported his findings with this blue light source in 40 individuals with mild to moderate inflammatory acne vulgaris. Treatments were conducted two times per week for 4 weeks, with follow-up at 1 and 4 months. The results of this trial showed a 43% improvement in inflammatory acne (Figs. 6.9, 6.10). A different blue light source has also been shown to be more effective than topical 1% clindamycin solution in treating inflammatory acne vulgaris during a 4-week treatment period with a 1-month follow-up time period (Gold 2004b).

A variety of IPLs are also being used for the treatment of acne vulgaris. The mechanism of

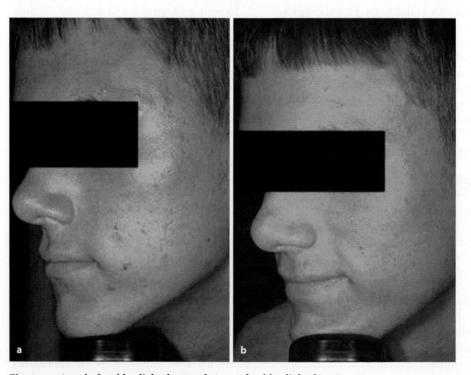

Fig. 6.9. a Acne before blue light therapy. **b** Acne after blue light therapy

action for IPL is similar to that seen with blue light therapy; that is, destruction of the *P. acnes* leading to a PDT effect. In one IPL study, 85% of patients showed greater than 50% improvement in their acne lesions. Unfortunately, 15%–20% of the patients were nonresponders.

Other investigators have looked at other laser systems whose primary effect may be the destruction of the sebaceous glands themselves. Lloyd and Mirkov (Lloyd and Mirkov 2002) evaluated the use of a 810-nm diode laser with application of indocyanin green. The indocyanin green is selectively absorbed into sebaceous glands and can be destroyed with exposure to the 810-nm diode laser. Paithanker et al. (Paithankar et al. 2002) have studied the 1450-nm laser for the treatment of inflammatory acne lesions. Their clinical evaluations have shown significant destructions of the sebaceous glands with this therapy and long-lasting resolution of the acne lesions.

Recently, a group of investigators has begun to evaluate the use of ALA as an enhancer for the laser and light therapies. Hongcharu et al.

(Hongcharu et al. 2000) looked at broadband light (500–700 nm) using ALA with a 3-h drug incubation period in 22 individuals. They noted significant clinical clearance 4 weeks after treatment which persisted up to 20 weeks. Adverse effects included an acneform folliculitis, postinflammatory hyperpigmentation, superficial peeling, and crusting. Itoh et al. (Itoh et al. 2000) reported on the use of ALA and a 635-nm pulsed excimer-dye laser in an intractable case of acne vulgaris on the face. The ALA was incubated for 4 h under occlusion. The treated area remained clear of acneform lesions during the 8-month follow-up period. A classic PDT reaction (erythema, edema, and crusting) was seen following the therapy. A second trial from Itoh et al. (Itoh et al. 2001) looked at a single ALA treatment in 13 individuals. Polychromatic visible light was used with a wavelength of 600–700 nm, 17 mW/cm², and 13 J/cm². The facial appearance of all the patients improved; new acne lesions were reduced at 1, 3, and 6 months after treatment. During the subsequent 6 months, acne lesions did reappear and seborrhea, reduced during

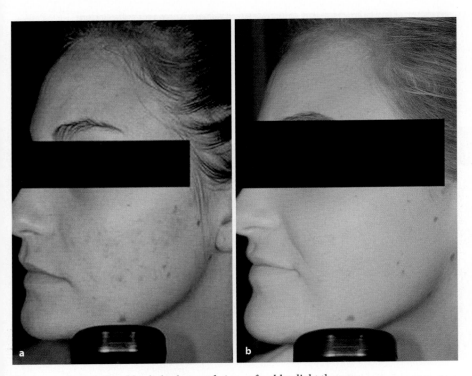

Fig. 6.10. **a** Acne before blue light therapy. **b** Acne after blue light therapy

therapy, also returned. Again, a classic PDT reaction occurred following the therapy with erythema, edema, and crusting noted in the patients following treatments.

Goldman (Goldman 2003) reported on the use of short-contact ALA-PDT with either IPL or a blue light device for the treatment of acne vulgaris and sebaceous gland hyperplasia. Treatments were noted to be pain free and without adverse effects. Relative clearing of the acne lesions were seen after 2–4 weekly treatments. Gold (Gold 2003) evaluated ten patients with moderate to severe acne vulgaris utilizing full-face, short-contact ALA-PDT and a high-intensity blue light source. Four weekly treatments showed a response of approximately 60% (versus 43% with the blue light source alone). Sessions were well tolerated with no noted adverse effects. Goldman and Boyce (Goldman 2003) also studied acne vulgaris with a blue light source with and without ALA in 22 individuals. Blue light therapy was performed alone twice per week for 2 weeks with a follow-up at 2 weeks; blue light plus ALA was performed two

times at 2-week intervals with a follow-up at 2 weeks after the final treatment. There was a greater response in the ALA-PDT/blue light group than blue light alone with no significant adverse effects seen in either group of patients. Gold (Gold 2004a) has now been evaluating a new IPL for moderate to severe acne vulgaris with ALA-PDT. Twenty patients were evaluated and results show significant improvement in inflammatory acne lesions; similar to previous studies performed by the author with blue light and ALA (Figs. 6.11, 6.12).

The combination of full-face, short-contact ALA-PDT treatments with blue light sources, IPLs, and other lasers and light sources appears to provide a synergistic effect to effectively treat patients suffering from moderate to severe inflammatory acne vulgaris. The combination therapy has been shown to be safe; it appears to work at a faster rate than lasers or light therapy alone, with fewer required treatments. This combination therapy may eliminate the need for more intensive systemic therapies in some of our patients.

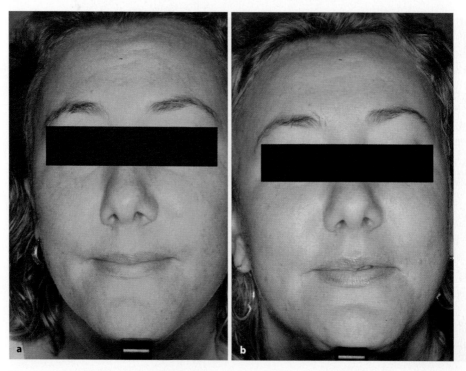

Fig. 6.11. **a** Acne before ALA-PDT/IPL therapy. **b** Acne after ALA-PDT/IPL therapy

■ Hidradenitis Suppurativa

Several other medical conditions are also being treated with ALA-PDT. Our group has recently reported on the successful use of ALA-PDT and a high-intensity blue light source in the treatment of hidradenitis suppurativa (HS). Four individu-als with recalcitrant HS were treated with short-contact ALA and between three and four sessions of the blue light source. The treatments were given at 1- to 2-week intervals. Seventy-five to one hundred percent of the HS lesions responded to this therapy and remained clear during a 3-month follow-up period. (Fig. 6.13).

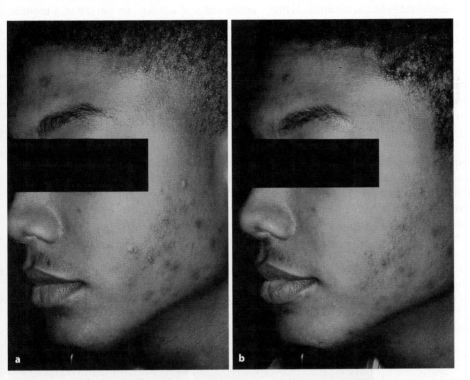

Fig. 6.12. **a** Acne before ALA-PDT/IPL therapy. **b** Acne after ALA-PDT/IPL therapy

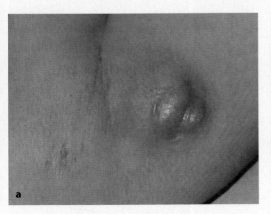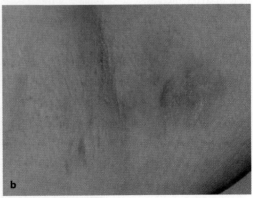

Fig. 6.13. **a** Hidradenitis suppurativa (HS) before ALA-PDT blue light therapy. **b** HS 3 months after ALA-PDT blue light therapy

■ Sebaceous Gland Hyperplasia

Sebaceous gland hyperplasia is an entity which has been treated with numerous therapeutic modalities. These have included cryotherapy, excision, electrodessication, laser vaporization, and oral isotretinoin use. These therapies are often associated with lesional recurrences or undesirable adverse side effects. Recently, Alster and Tanzi (Alster and Tanzi 2003) reported on the use of ALA and the 595-nm pulsed dye laser in the treatment of sebaceous gland hyperplasia lesions. Ten patients received short-contact ALA drug incubation (1 h) and one or two treatments at 6-week intervals. Results showed that seven individuals had clearing of the targeted sebaceous gland hyperplasia lesions with one ALA-pulsed dye laser treatment, and three patients required two treatments for lesion clearing. Follow-up in this group of patients was for 3 months. Matched lesions on the same patient served as controls; some were treated with pulsed dye laser and some not treated at all. The treatments were well tolerated by the study participants. Others have evaluated ten patients with short-contact ALA-PDT and the blue light source. Patients were given 3–6 weekly treatments and were followed for 6 months. Seventy percent of all lesions responded to therapy. Recurrence rates of up to 10–20% of lesions were seen within 3–4 months of the final treatment. Our group has also examined short-contact ALA-PDT in a group of patients who received either IPL therapy or a high-intensity blue light source. Results from 4 weekly treatments show both therapies useful in the treatment of sebaceous gland hyperplasia, with 50% of lesions responding during the treatment and a follow-up period of 3 months. (Fig. 6.14).

Advantages

ALA-PDT therapy is an important new treatment modality which enhances already proven and successful laser and light source treatments. It must be remembered that, at the time of this writing, the only FDA-approved indication for ALA-PDT is for the treatment of nonhyperkeratotic AKs on the face and scalp and treated with the blue light source after a 14- to 18-h drug incubation period. The clinical trials presented for photorejuvenation, acne vulgaris, HS, and sebaceous gland hyperplasia, and the methodology used by the investigators are all being performed as off-label clinical trials. Clinicians can use medicines in an off-label format; patients should be made aware of the off-label

Fig. 6.14.
a Sebaceous gland hyperplasia (SGH) before ALA-PDT/IPL therapy.
b SGH after ALA-PDT/IPL therapy

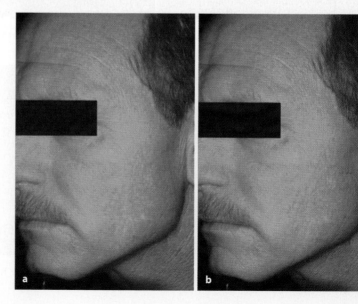

use of these treatments and proper informed consents should be made prior to the actual treatments (Figs. 6.15, 6.16). Research into entities being treated with ALA-PDT is growing and more investigations will follow in the months and years to come.

Psoriasis and Disorders of Hypopigmentation

■ Psoriasis Vulgaris

Psoriasis vulgaris is dermatologic disease which has recently been successfully treated with a new generation of lasers and light sources. Psoriasis is a chronic, noncontagious skin disease which affects between 1% and 3% of the population, or about 7 million people in the United States. It is the seventh most common reason patients seek

CONSENT FOR LEVULAN PHOTODYNAMIC TREATMENT

Levulan (Aminolevulinic acid 20%) is a naturally occurring photosensitizing compound which has been approved by the FDA and Health and Welfare Canada to treat pre-cancerous skin lesions called actinic keratosis. Levulan is applied to the skin and subsequently "activated" by specific wavelengths of light. This process of activating Levulan with light is termed Photodynamic Therapy. The purpose of activating the Levulan is to improve the appearance and reduce acne rosacea, acne vulgaris, sebaceous hyperplasia, decrease oiliness of the skin, and improve texture and smoothness by minimizing pore size. Any pre-cancerous lesions are also simultaneously treated. The improvement of these skin conditions (other than actinic keratosis) is considered an "off-label" use of Levulan.

I understand that Levulan will be applied to my skin for 30–60 minutes. Subsequently, the area will be treated with a specific wavelength of light to activate the Levulan. Following my treatment, I must wash off any Levulan on my skin. I understand that I should avoid direct sunlight for 24 hours following the treatment due to photosensitivity. I understand that I am not pregnant.

Anticipated side effects of Levulan treatment include discomfort, burning, swelling, blistering, scarring, redness and possible skin peeling, especially in any areas of sun damaged skin and pre-cancers of the skin, as well as lightening or darkening of skin tone and spots, and possible hair removal. The peeling may last many days, and the redness for several weeks if I have an exuberant response to treatment.

I consent to the taking of photographs of my face before each treatment session. I understand that I may require several treatment sessions spaced 1–6 weeks apart to achieve optimal results. I understand that I am responsible for payment of this procedure, as it is not covered by health insurance.

I understand that medicine is not an exact science, and that there can be no guarantees of my results. I am aware that while some individuals have fabulous results, it is possible that these treatments will not work for me. I understand that alternative treatments include topical medications, oral medications, cryosurgery, excisional surgery, and doing nothing.

I have read the above information and understand it. My questions have been answered satisfactorily by the doctor and his staff. I accept the risks and complications of the procedure. By signing this consent form I agree to have one or more Levulan treatments.

. . . .
Name   Signature

. . . .
Date   Witness

Fig. 6.15. Informed consent for ALA-PDT

CONSENT FOR ULTRAVIOLET LIGHT TYPE B-PHOTOTHERAPY

Phototherapy involves the exposure of the involved skin to a short-wave ultraviolet light known as UVB. UVB occurs naturally in sunlight; it is the part of the sunlight, which causes sunburns.

The dosage of UVB will be determined on many factors such as type of skin, disease, age, and type of equipment. The time is gradually increased until the desired result is achieved. At all times, while inside the phototherapy light box, special protective eyewear must be worn. Men will also protect their scrotum area.

The side effects to ultra-phototherapy B are, during treatment the psoriasis can sometimes get temporarily worse before getting better. The skin may itch and get red due to overexposure (sunburn). The long-term risk in developing skin cancer(s) from long-term exposure to UVB is unknown. Also, long-term exposure can cause freckling and loss of skin elasticity.

During the course of therapy, your skin will be evaluated.

6

Also, I agree that any pictures taken of me can be used for either teaching or publication unless I notify the staff in writing that they are not to use my pictures.

Fig. 6.16. Informed consent for laser/light therapy for psoriasis and disorders of hypopigmentation

dermatologic care. Numerous studies have noted significant quality of life issues in patients with psoriasis. Psoriasis varies in severity from mild to moderate to severe disease. Mild psoriasis vulgaris involves disease activity of less than 2% body surface area, moderate disease between 2% and 10%, and severe psoriasis generally involves greater than 10% body surface area. Genetics, biochemical pathways, and the immune system are known to be involved in the pathogenesis of psoriasis. In psoriasis, faulty immune signals are thought to accelerate the skin growth cycles. This leads to an increase in the amount of skin cells, which pile up on the skin surface faster than the body can shed them – in 3–4 days instead of the normal 28 days. Much of the recent evidence into the pathogenesis of psoriasis suggests that psoriasis is a T-cell-mediated disease.

A variety of treatment options exist for patients suffering from psoriasis. Most of the treatments are safe and effective. These treatments improve the psoriatic skin and reduce the symptoms associated with psoriasis, mainly swelling, erythema, flaking, and pruritis. These therapies (Table 6.3) often lead to a remission in the skin condition. A step-ladder approach to psoriasis therapy is commonly used by most clinicians. (Table 6.3). With this approach to the

Table 6.3. Treatment options for psoriasis vulgaris

Step 1: Topical Therapy
  Topical corticosteroids
  Topical coal tar
  Topical calcepotriene (Vitamin D)
  Topical vitamin A derivatives
  Topical anthralin
  Topical salicylic acid
  Natural sunlight

Step 2: Phototherapy/lasers
  Ultraviolet B (UVB) light
  Narrowband UVB
  B Clear (Lumenis)
  Xtrac (PhotoMedex) excimer laser
  PUVA (psoralen plus ultraviolet A light)

Step 3: Systemic medications
  Methotrexate
  Oral retinoids
  Cyclosporine
  Biologic drugs – alefacept (Amevive)
  Efalizumal (Raptiva)
  Etanercept (Enbrel)
  Infliximal (Remicade)

use of phototherapy, a variety of new lasers and light sources are being evaluated.

The major light sources being used for the treatment of psoriasis are the BClear (Lumenis) and the Xtrac (PhotoMedix). Clinical trials with the XTrac, a 308-nm excimer laser, have shown significant clearing of psoriatic plaques. Feldman et al. (Feldman et al. 2002) reported on a multicenter analysis with 124 patients at five centers. Seventy-two percent of patients demonstrated 75% or greater clearance in 6.2 treatments or less. Eighty-four percent achieved improvement of 75% or better after ten treatments. Other investigators also showed significant clearance using the excimer laser in 11 patients after 1 month of therapy; five patients remained disease free at a 4-month follow-up (Figs. 6.17, 6.18). The BClear is a narrowband UVB device which delivers the UVB in a focused, fiber-optic delivery system. This allows the UVB to be delivered only to diseased tissue, leaving healthy tissue alone. Such an approach leads to the potential for less treatment sessions. Potential adverse effects and the development of skin cancers may also be lessened. This device produces UVB light in the 290- to 320-nm range with most emitted wavelengths between 311 and 314 nm. The device may deliver light either in a single pulse mode or continuous pulse mode. Pulse widths of 0.5, 1.0, 1.5, and 2.0 s exist. Fluences range from 50 to 800 mJ and spot sizes up to 16×16 mm exist for the device. Several clinical trials have shown significant clearances with this targeted UVB system. (Figs. 6.19, 6.20).

■ **Vitiligo**

A variety of leukodermas of the skin have also been treated with both the excimer laser and targeted UVB systems. Leukodermas of the skin are defined as loss of skin pigment from a disease process (i. e., vitiligo) or secondary to an injury pattern to the skin (including loss of pigment from burns, surgical procedures, and following laser resurfacing procedures). Other skin concerns, such as idiopathic guttate hypomelanosis and hypopigmented stretch marks are also being evaluated with these technologies. Vitiligo is a pigmentation disorder in which

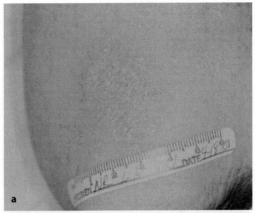
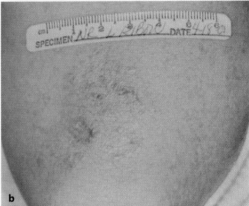
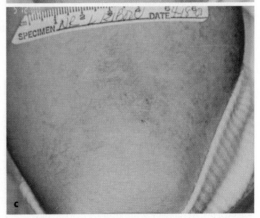

Fig. 6.17. **a** Psoriasis before excimer laser treatment. **b** Psoriasis after three excimer laser treatments. **c** Psoriasis after six excimer laser treatments

6

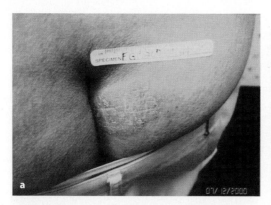 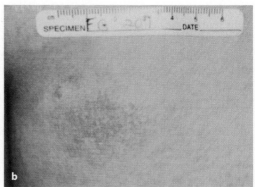

Fig. 6.18. **a** Psoriasis before excimer laser treatment. **b** Psoriasis after ten excimer laser treatments

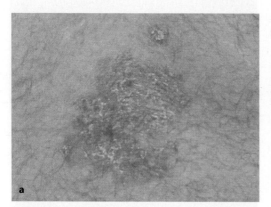 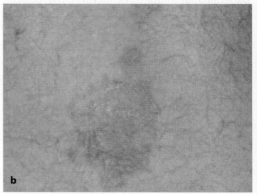

Fig. 6.19. **a** Psoriasis before narrowband UVB targeted therapy. **b** Psoriasis after ten narrowband UVB targeted therapy treatments

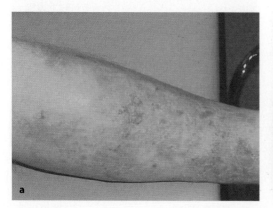 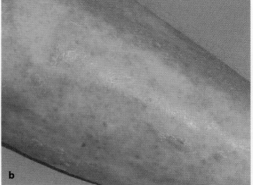

Fig. 6.20. **a** Psoriasis before narrowband UVB targeted therapy. **b** Psoriasis after ten narrowband UVB targeted therapy treatments

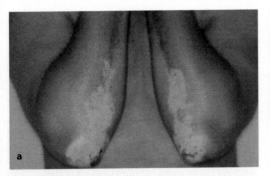 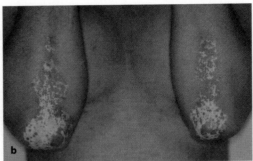

Fig. 6.21. **a** Vitiligo before excimer laser. **b** Vitiligo after ten excimer laser treatments

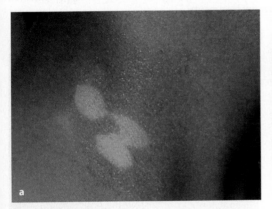 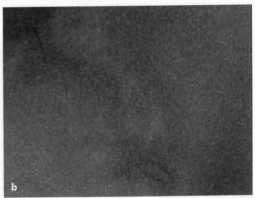

Fig. 6.22. **a** Vitiligo before narrowband UVB targeted therapy. **b** Vitiligo after four narrowband UVB targeted therapy treatments

melanocytes in the skin, mucous membranes, and the retina of the eye may be destroyed. As a result, white patches of skin can appear on different parts of the body. The cause of vitiligo is unknown; genetics may play a role and vitiligo is often associated with autoimmune diseases. Vitiligo affects between 1 and 2% of the world population, or between 40 and 50 million people worldwide. All races and both sexes are equally affected. A variety of therapies are available in an attempt to repigment those affected with vitiligo. The 308-nm excimer laser has shown promising results in the treatment of vitiligo. Spencer et al. (Spencer et al. 2002) evaluated 18 patients with vitiligo. Twenty three patches of vitiligo, in 12 patients, received at least six treatments with the excimer laser. A response rate of 57% was noted. Eleven patches, in six patients, received 12 treatments and had

an 82% response rate. (Fig. 6.21). A targeted narrowband UVB device can also be used for repigmentation. Initial clinical reports support its usefulness in the treatment of vitiligo (Fig. 6.22).

■ Hypopigmented Stretch Marks

Hypopigmented stretch marks (striae) are often seen in dermatologic and cosmetic clinics. Vascular stretch marks are easy to treat with a variety of vascular lasers and IPLs. Hypopigmented stretch marks are more difficult to treat. Goldberg and his group (Sarradet et al. 2002) treated ten patients with mature hypopigmented striae using the 308 nm excimer laser. Repigmentation was noted in all study participants; acceptable results were seen in 70% of the individuals. The targeted UVB device may improve this loss of

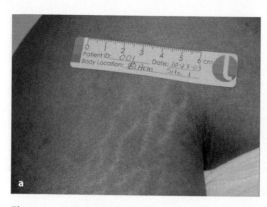 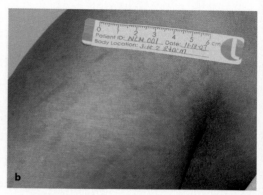

Fig. 6.23. **a** Hypopigmented stretch marks before narrowband UVB targeted therapy. **b** Hypopigmented stretch marks after four narrowband UVB targeted therapy treatments

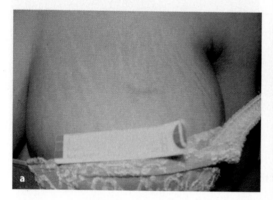 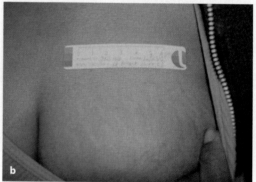

Fig. 6.24. **a** Hypopigmented stretch marks before narrowband UVB targeted therapy. **b** Hypopigmented stretch marks after four narrowband UVB targeted therapy treatments

pigmentation. We also have evaluated 50 individuals who after ten treatments were noted to have between 30 and 40% repigmentation. (Figs. 6.23, 6.24).

Disadvantages

The lasers and light sources used in the treatment of medical dermatologic skin concerns have a low incidence of adverse effects. The use of ALA-PDT can show a "PDT effect" generally described after prolonged drug incubation and exposure to light sources. This PDT effect of erythema, edema, and crusting has been shown to last up to 1 week after light exposure. It is less likely to occur with the use of full-face, short-contact therapy. Lasers and light sources can cause erythema, blisters, burns and, on occasion, scarring. No procedure is without an occasional complication.

The lasers and light sources being utilized for psoriasis vulgaris and disorders of hypopigmentation have shown themselves to be very safe and devoid of major complications.

Contraindications

Contraindications are rare when utilizing lasers and light sources for the treatment of medical dermatologic conditions with or without ALA-PDT. As with all laser and light treatments, patient expectations must be carefully addressed. Multiple treatments are often required to produce optimal results. Maintenance therapies will also be required in most instances.

Most laser physicians would not recommend the use of oral isotretinoin when performing laser and light treatments. Whether this is an absolute contraindication is open for debate, but caution should be used if oral isotretinoin is used during these laser or light procedures.

Personal Laser Technique

ALA-PDT Technique

The technique which we use varies depending upon the condition which is being treated. The two most common uses of ALA-PDT in our office setting are: (1) for photodynamic photorejuvenation, and (2) for the treatment of moderated to severe acne vulgaris. Both techniques are described below.

ALA-PDT for photodynamic photorejuvenation utilizes the Levulan Kerastick, and the following light sources: blue light, the intense pulsed light source, and/or the pulsed dye laser. The preparation prior to the procedure is the same for each device. The areas to be treated are cleansed with a mild facial cleanser. For increased penetration of the ALA, in those with moderate to severe actinic damage, a vigorous acetone scrub or a microdermabrasion procedure is performed prior to application of the ALA. The ALA is prepared as described above. ALA is applied to the entire area being treated in an even distribution and allowed to incubate for approximately 1-h prior to laser/light therapy. Before the procedure is performed, the ALA is washed off the face with a mild cleanser. The choice of light source is up to each practitioner – head to head clinical trials have not been performed to determine if one light source is superior to another; in my experience, all work well and deliver the desired results. We explain to our patients that treatments are performed once a month for up to four treatments, with the actual number determined by the patient's response to the therapy.

For the treatment of moderate to severe acne vulgaris, the procedures previously outlined are once again utilized. For our acne patients, we typically treat patients every other week for up to four visits, all dependent on the patient's response to the therapy.

■ Psoriasis Vulgaris and Disorders of Pigmentation Techniques

The two main light sources we currently utilize for psoriasis vulgaris and disorders of hypopigmentation are the narrowband UVB source and the excimer laser. Multiple therapies with each modality are required and maintenance therapies will be needed.

Postoperative Care

Postoperative Care Following ALA-PDT

Here are some care instructions for patients following ALA-PDT photodynamic skin rejuvenation.

■ On the Day of Treatment

1. If you have any discomfort, begin applying ice packs to the treated areas. This will help keep the area cool and alleviate any discomfort, as well as help keep down any swelling. Swelling will be most evident around the eyes and is usually more prominent in the morning.
2. Remain indoors and avoid direct sunlight.
3. Spray on Avene Thermal Spring Water often.
4. Apply Cetaphil moisturizing cream.
5. Take analgesics such as Advil if necessary.
6. If given any topical medications, apply twice daily to the treated area.

■ Days 2–7

1. You may begin applying make-up once any crusting has healed. The area may be slightly red for 1–2 weeks. If make-up is important to you, please see one of our aestheticians for a complimentary consultation.

2. The skin will feel dry and tightened. Cetaphil moisturizer should be used daily.
3. Try to avoid direct sunlight for 1 week. Use a total block Zinc Oxide based sunscreen with a minimum SPF 30.

Postoperative Care for Psoriasis and Disorders of Hypopigmentations

You have been treated with a UVB light source. Therefore, some redness may occur to the treated areas.

1. If redness occurs, you may use ice packs or aloe vera gel to the treated areas.
2. Avoid sunlight for the first couple of days after treatment. You may use sunscreen if you must be outdoors.

The Future

A variety of medical concerns are now being treated with lasers and light sources. The advent of ALA-PDT has heralded a potentially new era for dermatologists and laser surgeons far beyond the treatment of AKs, BCCs, and SCCs. Now "photodynamic photorejuvenation" is a common term and photorejuvenation treatments are being enhanced with the use of ALA-PDT. Other entities, including acne vulgaris, hidradenitis suppurativa, and sebaceous gland hyperplasia are being treated with lasers, light sources, and ALA-PDT. Lasers and light sources are also being used to treat psoriasis vulgaris, vitiligo, and other hypopigmented disorders, including hypopigmented stretch marks. Lasers and light sources can now be used to treat both medical and cosmetic dermatologic conditions.

References

Alexiades-Armenakas M, Geronemus R. (2003) Laser mediated photodynamic therapy of actinic keratoses. Arch Dermatol 139:1313–1320

Alster TS, Tanzi EL (2003) Photodynamic therapy with topical aminolevulinic acid and pulsed dye laser irradiation for sebaceous hyperplasia. J Drugs Dermatol 2(5):501–504

Avram D, Goldman MP (2004) Effectiveness and safety of ALA-IPL in treating actinic keratoses and photodamage. J Drugs Dermatol 3(5):36–39

Dougherty TJ, Kaufman JE (1978) Goldfarb A, et al. Photoradiation therapy for the treatment of malignant tumors. Cancer Res 38:2628–2635

Elman M, Slatkine M, Harth Y (2003) The effective treatment of acne vulgaris by a high-intensity, narrow band 405–420 nm light source. J Cosmet Laser Ther 5:111–117

Feldman SR, et al. (2002) Efficacy of 308 nm excimer laser for treatment of psoriasis: results of a multicenter study. J Am Acad Dermatol 46(6):900–906

Gold MH (2003) Intense pulsed light therapy for photorejuvenation enhanced with 20% aminolevulinic acid photodynamic therapy. J Laser Med Surg 15(Suppl):47

Gold, MH (2004a) A multi-center study of photodynamic therapy in the treatment of moderate to severe inflammatory acne vulgaris with topical 20% 5-aminolevulinic acid and a new intense pulsed light source. J Am Acad Derm 50(Suppl):54

Gold MH (2004b) A multi-center investigatory study of the treatment of mild to moderate inflammatory acne vulgaris of the face with visible blue light in comparison to topical 1% clindamycin antibiotic solution. J Am Acad Derm 50(Suppl):56

Gold MH, Bridges T, Bradshaw V, et al. (2004) ALA-PDT and blue light therapy for hidradenitis suppurativa. J Drugs Dermatol 3(Suppl):32–39

Goldman MP (2003) Using 5-aminolevulinic acid to treat acne and sebaceous hyperplasia. Cosmet Dermatol 16:57–58

Goldman MP, Atkin D, Kincad S (2002) PDT/ALA in the treatment of actinic damage: real world experience. J Laser Med Surg 14(Suppl):24

Goldman MP, Boyce S (2003) A single-center study of aminolevulinic acid and 417 nm photodynamic therapy in the treatment of moderate to severe acne vulgaris. J Drugs Dermatol 2:393–396

Hongcharu W, Taylor CR, Chang Y, et al. (2000) Topical ALA-photodynamic therapy for the treatment of acne vulgaris. J Invest Dermatol 115(2):183–192

Itoh Y, Ninomiya Y, Tajima S, Ishibashi A (2000) Photodynamic therapy for acne vulgaris with topical 5-aminolevulinic acid. Arch Dermatol 136(9):1093–1095

Itoh Y, Ninomiya Y, Tajima S, et al. (2001) Photodynamic therapy of acne vulgaris with topical delta aminolevulinic acid and incoherent light in Japanese patients. Br J Dermatol 144:575–579

Kalka K, et al. (2000) Photodynamic therapy in dermatology. J Am Acad Dermatol 42:389–413

Lloyd JR, Mirkov M (2002) Selective photothermolysis of the sebaceous glands for acne treatment. Lasers Surg Med 31:115–120

Lui H, Anderson RR (1993) Photodynamic therapy in dermatology: recent developments. Dermatol Clin 11:1–13

Paithankar DY, Ross EV, Saleh BA, Blair MA, Graham BS (2002) Acne treatment with a 1,450 nm wavelength laser and cryogen spray cooling. Lasers Surg Med 31:106–114

Papageorgiou P, et al. (2000) Phototherapy with blue (415 nm) and red (660 nm) light in the treatment of acne vulgaris. Br J Dermatol 142:973–978

Rowe PM (1988) Photodynamic therapy begins to shine. Lancet 351:1496

Ruiz-Rodriquez R, Sanz-Sanchez T, Cordobo S (2002) Photodynamic photorejuvenation. Dermatol Surg 28:742–744

Sarradet D, Hussein M, Solana LG, Goldberg DJ (2002) Repigmentation of striae with a 308 nm excimer laser. Lasers Med Surg 14(Suppl):44–45

Sigurdsson V, et al. (1997) Phototherapy of acne vulgaris with visible light. Dermatology 194:256–260

Spencer JM, Nossa R, Ajmeri J (2002) Treatment of vitiligo with the 308 nm excimer laser: a pilot study. J Am Acad Dermatol 40:727–731

Svassand LO, et al. (1996) Light and drug distribution with topically administered photosensitizers. Lasers Med Surg 11:261–265

Velicer CM, et al. (2004) Antibiotic use in relation to the risk of breast cancer. JAMA 291:827–835

Subject Index